WORLD HEALTH ORGANIZATION

CORRIGENDA

ENVIRONMENTAL HEALTH CRITERIA
NO. 102

1-PROPANOL

Page 2, line 14:
Delete: 1.1-Propanol
Insert: 1.Alcohol, propyl

Page 2, line 15:
Delete: QV 223
Insert: QD 305.A4

Environmental Health Criteria 102

1-PROPANOL

Published under the joint sponsorship of
the United Nations Environment Programme,
the International Labour Organisation,
and the World Health Organization

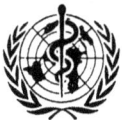

World Health Organization
Geneva, 1990

The International Programme on Chemical Safety (IPCS) is a joint venture of the United Nations Environment Programme, the International Labour Organisation, and the World Health Organization. The main objective of the IPCS is to carry out and disseminate evaluations of the effects of chemicals on human health and the quality of the environment. Supporting activities include the development of epidemiological, experimental laboratory, and risk-assessment methods that could produce internationally comparable results, and the development of manpower in the field of toxicology. Other activities carried out by the IPCS include the development of know-how for coping with chemical accidents, coordination of laboratory testing and epidemiological studies, and promotion of research on the mechanisms of the biological action of chemicals.

WHO Library Cataloguing in Publication Data

1-Propanol

(Environmental health criteria ; 102)

1.1-Propanol   I.Series

ISBN 92 4 157102 0   (NLM Classification: QV 223)
ISSN 0250-863X

Computer typesetting by HEADS, Oxford OX7 2NY, England

PRINTED IN FINLAND
Vammalan Kirjapaino Oy
89/000 — VAMMALA — 0000

CONTENTS

3

WHO TASK GROUP MEETING ON ENVIRONMENTAL HEALTH CRITERIA FOR 1-PROPANOL

Members

Dr R. Drew, Department of Clinical Pharmacology, Flinders University of South Australia, Bedford Park, South Australia, Australia

Dr B. Gilbert, Company for Development of Technology Transfer (CODETEC), City University, Campinas, Brazil (*Rapporteur*)

Dr B. Hardin, Document Development Branch, Division of Standards Development and Technology Transfer, National Institute for Occupational Safety and Health, Cincinnati, Ohio, USA (*Chairman*)

Dr S.K. Kashyap, National Institute of Occupational Health, Ahmedabad, India

Professor M. Noweir, Occupational Health Research Centre, High Institute of Public Health, University of Alexandria, Alexandria, Egypt

Dr L. Rosenstein, Office of Toxic Substances, US Environmental Protection Agency, Washington, DC, USA

Professor I.V. Sanotsky, Chief, Department of Toxicology Institute of Industrial Hygiene and Occupational Diseases, Moscow, USSR (*Vice-Chairman*)

Dr J. Sokal, Division of Industrial Toxicology, Institute of Occupational Medicine, Lodz, Poland

Dr H.J. Wiegand, Toxicology Department, Huls AG, Marl, Federal Republic of Germany

Dr K. Woodward, Department of Health, Medical Toxicology and Environmental Health Division, London, United Kingdom

Observers

Dr K. Miller (Representing International Commission on Occupational Health (ICOH)), British Industrial Biological Research Association, Carshalton, Surrey, United Kingdom

Secretariat

Professor F. Valić, Consultant, IPCS, World Health Organization, Geneva, Switzerland, *also* Vice-Rector, University of Zagreb, Zagreb, Yugoslavia (*Secretary*)

Dr T. Vermeire, National Institute of Public Health and Environmental Hygiene, Bilthoven, Holland

Host Organization

Dr S.D. Gangolli, British Industrial Biological Research Association, Carshalton, Surrey, United Kingdom

Dr D. Anderson, British Industrial Biological Research Association, Carshalton, Surrey, United Kingdom

NOTE TO READERS OF THE CRITERIA DOCUMENTS

Every effort has been made to present information in the criteria documents as accurately as possible without unduly delaying their publication. In the interest of all users of the environmental health criteria documents, readers are kindly requested to communicate any errors that may have occurred to the Manager of the International Programme on Chemical Safety, World Health Organization, Geneva, Switzerland, in order that they may be included in corrigenda, which will appear in subsequent volumes.

* * *

A detailed data profile and a legal file can be obtained from the International Register of Potentially Toxic Chemicals, Palais des Nations, 1211 Geneva 10, Switzerland (Telephone no. 7988400/ 7985850).

ENVIRONMENTAL HEALTH CRITERIA FOR 1-PROPANOL

A WHO Task Group on Environmental Health Criteria for 1-Propanol met at the British Industrial Biological Research Association (BIBRA), Carshalton, Surrey, United Kingdom, from 10 to 14 April 1989. Dr S.D. Gangolli, who opened the meeting, welcomed the participants on behalf of the Department of Health, and Dr D. Anderson on behalf of BIBRA, the host institution. Dr F. Valic greeted the participants on behalf of the heads of the three IPCS cooperating organizations (UNEP/ILO/WHO). The Task Group reviewed and revised the draft criteria document and made an evaluation of the human health risks and effects on the environment of exposure to 1-propanol.

The drafts of this document were prepared by Dr T. VERMEIRE, National Institute of Public Health and Environmental Hygiene, Bilthoven, Netherlands. Dr F. VALIC was responsible for the overall scientific content of the document and Mrs M.O. HEAD of Oxford, England, for the editing.

The efforts of all who helped in the preparation and finalization of the document are gratefully acknowledged.

* * *

Partial financial support for the publication of this criteria document was kindly provided by the United States Department of Health and Human Services, through a contract from the National Institute of Environmental Health Sciences, Research Triangle Park, North Carolina, USA — a WHO Collaborating Centre for Environmental Health Effects. The United Kingdom Department of Health and Social Security generously supported the cost of printing.

1. SUMMARY

1.1. Identity, Physical and Chemical Properties, Analytical Methods

1-Propanol is a colourless, highly flammable liquid that is volatile at room temperature and normal atmospheric pressure. It is miscible with water and organic solvents. Analytical methods for propanol include gas chromatography, which can detect 5×10^{-5} mg/m^3 in air, 1×10^{-4} mg/litre in water, and 0.002 mg/litre in blood, serum, or urine, when suitable extraction or concentration procedures are used with the sample.

1.2 Sources of Human and Environmental Exposure

The annual world production capacity in 1979 exceeded 130 000 tonnes. It is produced in nature by the decomposition of organic materials by a variety of microorganisms, and occurs in plants and fuel oil. 1-Propanol is produced from ethene by reaction with carbon monoxide and hydrogen to give propionaldehyde, which is then hydrogenated. It is also a by-product of methanol manufacture and may be produced from propane directly or from acrolein. The major use of 1-propanol is as a multi-purpose solvent in industry and in the home. It is used in flexographic printing ink and textile applications, products for personal use, such as cosmetics and lotions, and in window cleaning, polishing, and antiseptic formulations. Second in importance is its use as an intermediate in the manufacture of a variety of chemical compounds.

1.3. Environmental Transport, Distribution and Transformation

The main pathway of entry of 1-propanol into the environment is through its emission into the atmosphere during production, processing, storage, transport, use, and waste disposal. Emissions into water and soil also occur. Because the main use of 1-propanol is as a volatile solvent, much of the production volume is eventually released into the environment.

1-Propanol rapidly disappears from the atmosphere by reaction with hydroxyl radicals and through rain-out. It is readily

11

biodegradable, both aerobically and anaerobically, and, because of these chemical and biological removal mechanisms, measurable levels are not normally encountered in the environment. However, the compound has been detected in urban air, at waste-disposal sites, and also in water leaching from a landfill. Soil permeability for 1-propanol is probably high and the compound enhances permeability for some aromatic solvents.

1-Propanol has a log *n*-octanol/water partition coefficient of 0.34 and a bioconcentration factor of 0.7, which render bioaccumulation highly unlikely.

1.4 Environmental Levels and Human Exposures

Exposure of the general population may occur through accidental ingestion, through inhalation during use, and through ingestion via food (containing 1-propanol as a natural or added flavour volatile or as a solvent residue) and non-alcoholic as well as alcoholic beverages. For example, beer contains up to 195 mg/litre, wine up to 116 mg/litre, and various types of spirit up to 3520 mg/litre. Exposure of the general population to 1-propanol via inhalation and drinking-water is low (in the USA the average concentration in urban air samples was 0.00005 mg/m^3 and that in drinking-water, 0.001 mg/litre). Workers are potentially exposed through inhalation during manufacture, processing, and use. However, no data are available to quantify such exposures.

1.5 Kinetics and Metabolism

1-Propanol is rapidly absorbed and distributed throughout the body following ingestion. Data on the absorption rate following inhalation and dermal exposures are lacking. 1-Propanol is metabolized by alcohol dehydrogenase (ADH) to propionic acid via the aldehyde and may enter the tricarboxylic acid cycle. This oxidation is a rate-limiting step of 1-propanol metabolism. *In vitro*, rat and rabbit microsomal oxidases are also capable of oxidizing 1-propanol to propionic aldehyde. The relative affinity of ADH and the microsomal oxidizing systems for 1-propanol is much higher than that of ethanol; therefore 1-propanol is rapidly eliminated from the organism. In the rat, the half-life after an oral dose of 1000 mg/kg was 45 min.

In both animals and man, 1-propanol may be eliminated from the body in the expired air or in urine. In human beings administered an oral dose of 1-propanol of 3.75 mg/kg body weight and 1200 mg ethanol/kg body weight, the total urinary excretion of 1-propanol was 2.1% of the dose. The urinary levels of 1-propanol were lower the lower the amount of simultaneously ingested ethanol, showing competition for ADH between 1-propanol and the ethanol overdose.

1.6 Effects on Organisms in the Environment

At concentrations normally encountered in the environment, 1-propanol is not toxic for aquatic organisms, insects, or plants. The inhibitory threshold for cell multiplication of three of the more sensitive aquatic species (3 protozoa) was 38–568 mg/litre. For the higher organisms, the lethal concentration was about 5000 mg/litre, varying remarkably little from one phylum to another and exhibiting a very steep dose–response curve. Some bacteria and micro-organisms in waste-water and activated sludge are able to adapt to concentrations greater than 17 000 mg/litre.

Seed germination may be inhibited or stimulated by 1-propanol depending on the concentration in water used and conditions of exposure. The compound increases nitrite accumulation in maize, peas, and wheat.

1.7 Effects on Experimental Animals and *In Vitro* Test Systems

The acute toxicity of 1-propanol for mammals (based on mortality) is low, whether exposure is via the dermal, oral, or the respiratory route. Oral LD_{50} values for several animal species have been reported to range between 1870 and 6800 mg/kg body weight. However, an oral LD_{50} of 560–660 mg/kg body weight was reported for very young rats. The principal toxic effect of 1-propanol following a single exposure is depression of the central nervous system. The available evidence for 1-propanol suggests that its effects on the central nervous system are similar to those of ethanol; however, 1-propanol appears to be more neurotoxic. The ED_{50} values for narcosis in rabbits and loss of righting reflex in mice were, respectively, 1440 mg/kg body weight orally, and 1478 mg/kg body weight intraperitoneally; these are approximately four times lower than those for ethanol. In the tilted plane test, 1-propanol was 2.5 times as potent as ethanol in rats.

Single oral doses of 3000 or 6000 mg/kg body weight resulted in a reversible accumulation of triglycerides in the liver of rats. High vapour concentrations caused irritation of the respiratory tract in mice. The respiratory rate in mice was decreased by 50% at concentrations of approximately 30 000 mg/m^3.

Data on eye and skin irritation are not available. No sensitization was observed in one reported skin sensitization test on CF1 mice.

There was limited evidence, in male rats exposed for 6 weeks to 15 220 mg/m^3, that 1-propanol impairs reproductive function. No effect was noted after a similar exposure to 8610 mg/m^3. When pregnant rats were exposed to 1-propanol, maternal and developmental toxicity were evident at 23 968 and 14 893 mg/m^3 (9743 and 6054 ppm); there was no toxicity at 9001 mg/m^3 (3659 ppm). No evidence was seen of behavioural defects in the offspring of male rats exposed for 6 weeks to 8610 or 15 220 mg 1-propanol/m^3, or in offspring of rats exposed during pregnancy to the same concentrations. However, when 5 to 8-day-old rats were orally dosed with 3000–7800 mg 1-propanol/kg, per day, there was evidence of CNS depression during dosing and signs of withdrawal when dosing ended. The brains of these rats were examined when they were 18 days old; reductions were found in the absolute and relative brain weights and in the contents of DNA as well as regional decreases in cholesterol and protein levels.

1-Propanol gave negative results in 2 assays for point mutations using *Salmonella typhimurium* and in a reverse mutation test with *Escherichia coli* CA-274. Negative results were obtained in tests for the induction of sister chromatid exchange or micronuclei in mammalian cells *in vitro*. No other mutagenicity data were available.

In a carcinogenicity study on small groups of Wistar rats exposed throughout their lifetime to oral doses of 240 mg/kg or to subcutaneous doses of 48 mg/kg, a significant increase in the incidence of liver sarcoma was noted in the group dosed subcutaneously. However, the study was inadequate for the assessment of carcinogenicity for a number of reasons including lack of experimental detail, too few animals, and the use of a high single dose inducing liver toxicity.

1.8 Health Effects on Human Beings

There are no reports of adverse health effects in the general population or in occupational groups. In the only fatal poisoning case reported, it was recorded that a woman was found unconscious and died 4–5 h after ingestion. Autopsy revealed a "swollen brain" and lung oedema. In a study on skin irritation and sensitization, allergic reactions were reported in a laboratory worker. In another group of 12 volunteers, erythema lasting for at least 60 min was observed in 9 individuals following a 5-min application of filter papers containing 0.025 ml of a 75% solution of 1-propanol in water on the forearms. No other reports on adverse health effects following occupational exposure to 1-propanol are available.

No epidemiological studies are available to assess the long-term effects, including the carcinogenicity, of 1-propanol in human beings.

1.9 Summary of Evaluation

Exposure of human beings to 1-propanol may occur through the ingestion of food or beverages containing 1-propanol. Inhalation exposure may occur during household use and occupationally during manufacture, processing, and use. The very limited data on the level of 1-propanol in the ambient air and water suggest that concentrations are very low.

1-Propanol is rapidly absorbed and distributed throughout the body following ingestion. Absorption following inhalation is expected to be rapid and dermal absorption is expected to be slow.

The acute toxicity of 1-Propanol for animals is low whether exposed via the dermal, oral, or the respiratory route. Exposure of members of the general population to potentially lethal levels may occur through accidental or intentional ingestion. However, only one case of lethal poisoning by 1-propanol has been reported. The most likely acute effects of 1-propanol in man are alcoholic intoxication and narcosis. The results of animal studies indicate that 1-propanol is 2–4 times as intoxicating as ethanol.

1-Propanol may be irritating to hydrated skin.

Animal toxicity data are not adequate to make an evaluation of the human health risks associated with repeated or long-term exposure to 1-propanol. However, limited short-term rat studies suggest that oral exposure to 1-propanol is unlikely to pose a serious health hazard under the usual conditions of human exposure.

Inhalation exposure to a concentration of 15 220 mg/m^3 caused impaired reproductive performance in male rats, but exposure to 8610 mg/m^3 did not. In pregnant rats, 9001 mg/m^3 (3659 ppm) was a no-observed-effect level (NOEL) and 14 893 mg/m^3 (6054 ppm) was a lowest-observed-effect level (LOEL) for both maternal and developmental toxicity. Thus, inhalation exposure to high concentrations of 1-propanol produced reproductive and developmental toxicity in male and female rats in the presence of overt toxicity in the exposed animals. The concentrations required to produce these effects in rats were higher than those likely to be encountered under normal conditions of human exposure.

1-Propanol was negative in assays for point mutations in bacteria. Although these findings suggest that the substance does not have any genotoxic potential, an adequate assessment of mutagenicity cannot be made on the basis of the limited data available. The available study is inadequate to evaluate the carcinogenicity of 1-propanol in experimental animals. No data are available on the long-term exposure of human populations to 1-propanol. Hence the carcinogenicity of 1-propanol for human beings cannot be evaluated.

Apart from one case of fatal poisoning following ingestion of half a litre of 1-propanol, there are practically no reports on the adverse health effects from exposure to 1-propanol, either in the general population or in occupational groups. The Task Group considers it unlikely that 1-propanol will pose a serious health risk for the general population under normal exposure conditions.

1-Propanol can be released into the environment during production, processing, storage, transport, use, and waste disposal. Because of its primary use as a volatile solvent, most of the production volume is eventually released into the atmosphere. However, by reacting with hydroxyl radicals and through rain-out, 1-propanol will disappear rapidly from the atmosphere, with a residence time of less than 3 days. Removal of 1-propanol from water and soil also occurs rapidly so that measurable levels are rarely found in any of the three compartments. Adsorption of 1-propanol on soil particles is poor, but it is mobile in soil and it has been shown to increase the permeability of soil to some aromatic hydrocarbons.

In view of the physical properties of 1-propanol, bioaccumulation is unlikely and, except in the case of accident or inappropriate disposal, 1-propanol does not present a risk for aquatic organisms, insects, and plants at concentrations that usually occur in the environment.

2. IDENTITY, PHYSICAL AND CHEMICAL PROPERTIES, ANALYTICAL METHODS

2.1 Identity

Chemical formula:	C_3H_8O
Chemical structure:	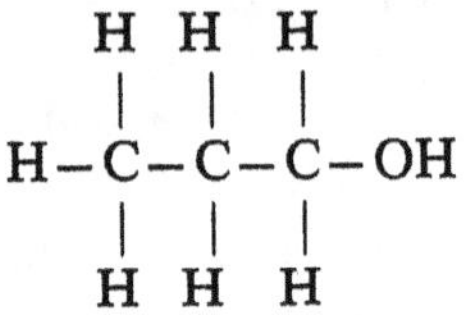
Common name:	*n*-propyl alcohol
Abbreviation:	NPA
Common synonyms:	ethyl carbinol, 1-hydroxypropane, propanol, *n*-propanol (IUPAC name), 1-propanol (CAS name), propan-1-ol
Common trade names:	Albacol, Optal, Osmosol extra, UN 1274
CAS registry number:	71-23-8
Specifications:	commercial 1-propanol contains typically 99.85% of the compound and, as main impurities, water ($\leq$ 0.1% by weight), aldehydes ($\leq$ 0.2% by weight), ethanol ($\leq$ 10 mg/kg), and methanol ($\leq$ 100 mg/kg) [35, 104–84).
Conversion factors:	1 ppm 1-propanol = 2.46 mg/m^3 air ; and 1 mg 1-propanol/m^3 air = 0.41 ppm, at 25 $^\circ$C and 101.3 kPa (760 mmHg).

2.2 Physical and Chemical Properties

1-Propanol is a highly flammable, volatile, colourless liquid at room temperature and standard atmospheric pressure. Its odour is described as alcohol-like, sweet, and pleasant [83]. Continuous exposure can result in loss of sensitivity to the odour (olfactory adaptation) [182]. The compound is completely miscible with water and with most organic solvents. It undergoes all chemical reactions typical of primary alcohols. 1-Propanol reacts violently with oxidizing agents.

Some physical and chemical data on 1-propanol are given in Table 1.

Table 1. Some physical and chemical properties of 1-propanol

Physical state	liquid
Colour	colourless
Relative molecular mass:	60.09
Odour perception threshold	< 0.07–100 mg/m^3 [a]
Odour recognition threshold	0.32–150 mg/m^3 [b]
Melting point (°C)	−127
Boiling point (°C)	97
Water solubility	infinite
Log *n*-octanol/water partition coefficient	0.34 [c]
Specific density (20 °C)	0.804
Relative vapour density	2.07
Vapour pressure (20 °C)	1.9 kPa (14.5 mmHg)
Flash point	
(open cup)	25 °C
(closed cup)	15 °C
Flammability limits	2.1–13.5% by volume

[a] From: May [122]; Corbit & Engen [42]; Oelert & Florian [138]; Stone et al. [182]; Dravnieks [50]; Hellman & Small [83]; Laing [111]; and Punter [151].
[b] From: May [122] and Hellman & Small [83].
[c] Experimentally derived by Hansch & Anderson [80].

2.3 Analytical Methods

A summary of methods for the determination of 1-propanol in air, water, and biological media is presented in Table 2.

Table 2. Sampling and analysis of 1-propanol

Medium	Sampling method	Analytical method	Detection limit	Sample size	Comments	Reference
Air	sampling on charcoal, desorption by carbon disulfide	gas chromatography with flame ionization detection	0.01 mg/sample	1–10 litre	suitable for personal and area monitoring; working range, 50–900 mg/m^3	[195]
Air	sampling on charcoal, desorption by a 1:1 mixture of carbon disulfide and water	gas chromatography with flame ionization detection, packed with Oronite NIW on Carbopack B	0.25 mg/m^3	24 litre	suitable for area monitoring, applicable mixtures of both polar and non-polar solvents	[112]
Air	condensation, pre-concentration by micro-distillation, purging by nitrogen, trapping on porous polymer, desorption by heating	gas chromatography with flame ionization detection, packed with Poropack QS and S	5×10^{-5} mg/m^3		suitable for analysis of oxygenated organic compounds in ambient air	[174]
Water	concentration by micro-distillation, purging by nitrogen, trapping on porous polymer, desorption by heating	gas chromatography with flame ionization detection, packed with Poropack QS and S	0.0001 mg/litre	60 ml	suitable for analysis of oxygenated organic compounds in water	[174]
Water	direct injection	gas chromatography with flame ionization detection, packed with porous polymer Tenax GC	1 mg/litre	0.001 ml	suitable for analysis of a mixture of a wide variety of compounds	[106]

Table 2. (contd).

Water	direct injection	gas chromatography with steam as carrier and flame ionization detection, packed with Chromosorb P AW modified with phosphoric acid	0.04 mg/ litre	0.002 ml	suitable for analysis of a mixture of aliphatic compounds	[194]
Water	derivatization by 2-fluoro-1-methyl-pyridinium p-toluene sulfonate in presence of tridodecylamine	paper electrophoresis with detection by Dragendorff's reagent	40 mg/ litre	0.1 ml	suitable for analysis of mixtures of primary and secondary alcohols, such as in alcoholic beverages	[8]
Water	derivatization with 4-(6-methylbenzo-thiazol-2-yl)phenyl isocyanate in presence of triethylene-diamine in xylene	TLC (silicagel G) or HPTLC (RP-18) or HPLC (Silicagel Si 60 or Li-Chrosorb RP-18) with fluorimetric detection	0.05 mg/ litre (TLC)	0.005 ml		[208]
Water	direct application	spot test detection using 0.1% vanadium(V)-N-phenylbenzohydroxa-mate in alcohol-free chloroform	2.5×10^{-2} mg/drop		a qualitative method with interference by other alcohols, phenols, cresols, dioxane, methylisobutyl ketone, acetone, reaction is immediate	[162]

21

Table 2 (contd).

Medium	Sampling method	Analytical method	Detection limit	Sample size	Comments	Reference
Serum, urine	extraction by dichloromethane	gas chromatography with mass spectrometric detection, column was coated with Emulphor ON-870	0.002 mg/litre	1 ml	suitable for determination of aliphatic alcohols	[114]
Blood, urine, tissue	addition of potassium carbonate; headspace sampling	gas chromatography with flame ionization detection; split columns packed with polypropylene glycol on Chromosorb W NAW and SP1000 on Carbopack, respectively	0.01 mg/litre	1.1 ml	whole blood is pretreated with sodium fluoride or perchloric acid; the method is applicable to tissue after equilibration with water	[21, 13, 110]
Blood	addition of sodium sulfate; headspace sampling	gas chromatography with flame ionization detection, split fused silica columns: DB 1701 and CP Sil 8 CB	0.01 mg/litre	0.1 ml		[209]

22

The sensitivity of the gas chromatographic determination of alcohols with electron capture or photoionization detection can be greatly improved by prior derivatization with pentafluorophenyl-dimethylsilyl chloride [109].

Ramsey & Flanagan [154] reported a method for the detection and identification of 1-propanol and other volatile organic compounds in the headspace of blood, plasma, or serum, using gas chromatography with flame ionization and electron capture detection. The method is applicable to samples obtained from victims of poisoning, for which a high sensitivity is not desirable. After preincubation of the samples with a proteolytic enzyme, the method can be used for the analysis of tissues.

Gas chromatographic methods, using flame ionization detection, are available for the determination of 1-propanol in milk and milk products [142], in alcoholic beverages [91, 71, 64, 148], in foodstuffs [148], in food packaging [54], in digestive contents, silage juices, and microorganism growth cultures [98], and in drug raw materials [121]. Methods for the identification of 1-propanol as flavour volatile have also been described (see Table 4, section 5.2).

3. SOURCES OF HUMAN AND ENVIRONMENTAL EXPOSURE

3.1 Natural Occurrence

1-propanol occurs in fuel oils. It has been identified as a metabolic product of microorganisms and as a flavour volatile in foodstuffs (section 5)[104]. Other potential sources of atmospheric alcohols are photochemical reactions of hydrocarbons, combustion, and, perhaps, oceans [174].

3.2 Man-Made Sources

3.2.1 Production levels and processes

The global capacity for the production of 1-propanol in 1979 exceeded 130 000 tonnes with most of this capacity in the USA [104]. In 1975, the total USA production amounted to 57 000 tonnes, and 6600 tonnes were exported [176]. In 1979, 85 000 tonnes were produced [104]. The production in the countries of the European Economic Community was estimated at 5100 tonnes in 1979 and 3300 tonnes over the first 9 months of 1983. The imports from the USA rose from 4000 tonnes in 1979 to 8700 tonnes over the first 9 months of 1983 [5]. 1-Propanol was not manufactured in eastern Europe or in the Far East in 1979, but one company in Japan was reported to produce this compound by Kirk & Othmer [104]

1-Propanol is manufactured by the hydroformylation of ethene (reaction with carbon monoxide and hydrogen) to propion-aldehyde, which is subsequently hydrogenated to 1-propanol [104]. The compound can also be recovered commercially as a by-product of the high pressure synthesis of methanol from carbon monoxide and hydrogen [35]. It has been produced by the vapour-phase oxidation of propane [104] and during the reduction of propene-derived acrolein [4, 35]. Earlier, 1-propanol was fractionally distilled from the fuel oils that form in the yeast fermentation process for the manufacture of ethanol [35].

3.2.2 Uses

The major use of 1-propanol is as a solvent. It is used as carrier and extraction solvent for natural products, such as flavourings, vegetable oils, resins, waxes, and gums, and as a solvent for synthetic polymers, such as polyvinyl butyral, cellulose esters, lacquers, and PVC adhesives. Other solvent applications include the use of 1-propanol in the polymerization and spinning of acrylonitrile, in flexographic printing inks, and in the dyeing of wool. 1-Propanol is used for both its solvent and antiseptic properties in drugs and cosmetics, such as lotions, soaps, and nail polishes. It is also used as a chemical intermediate, e.g., in the manufacture of propanal, 1-bromopropane, *O,O*-dipropylphosphoro- dithioic acid, *n*-propyl amines, esters (propyl acetate, propyl carbamate), alcoholates, and xanthates.

Miscellaneous uses include the application of 1-propanol in degreasing agents, polishing compounds (window cleaners, floor polishes), and brake fluid, as coupling and dispersing agents, and as a ruminant feed supplement. It improves the water tolerance of motor fuels [82, 104, 35, 198].

3.2.3 Waste disposal

1-Propanol may enter the atmosphere, water, and/or soil following waste disposal (section 4.1). At landfill sites, 1-propanol has been identified in the air and leachates (section 5.1). Emission of 1-propanol via waste gases and waste water occurs in industry, and diffuse airborne emissions occur during the use of the compound (section 4.1).

1-Propanol can be removed from waste water by biodegradation (section 4.3.1). Activated carbon adsorption is not feasible, because the compound is poorly adsorbed [69]. Removal of the compound from waste water by reverse osmosis (hyperfiltration) may be successful, depending on the type of membrane. Cellulose acetate membranes yielded an average of 40% separation of 1-propanol [53], while cross-linked polyethyleneimine membranes yielded 60–85% separation for a primary alcohol, such as ethanol [55]. Ozonization of 1-propanol appears to be too slow a process to be of any significance for water treatment [90].

4. ENVIRONMENTAL TRANSPORT, DISTRIBUTION, AND TRANSFORMATION

4.1 Transport and Distribution Between Media

In view of the physical properties and the use pattern of 1-propanol, it can be concluded that the main pathway of entry of this compound into the environment is through its emission into the atmosphere during production, handling, storage, transport, and use, and following waste disposal. Second in importance is its emission into water and soil. In the USA, industrial losses into the environment were estimated at 1.5% of the production in 1976, and 75% of the 1-propanol produced was estimated to be eventually released into the atmosphere [49].

Intercompartmental transfer of 1-propanol can occur between water, soil or waste, and air, and between soil or waste and water. Volatilization of the compound will be considerable in view of its rather high vapour pressure. Transport of 1-propanol from the atmosphere to soil or water will occur via rain-out, as it is highly soluble in water. Data on the behaviour of 1-propanol in soil are scarce. With respect to adsorption, there is one study showing that the compound is poorly adsorbed on activated carbon (198). Since 1-propanol is completely miscible with water, it can be expected to be mobile in the soil. It has also been shown to increase the permeability of soil to aromatic hydrocarbons [57].

4.2 Abiotic Degradation

Once in the atmosphere, 1-propanol is mainly degraded by hydroxyl radicals. It is not expected to react at appreciable rates with other reactive species, such as ozone, and hydroperoxy-, alkyl-, and alkoxy-radicals. Since the compound does not absorb ultraviolet radiation within the solar spectrum, photodegradation is not expected [34]. Experimentally determined rate constants for the reaction between 1-propanol and hydroxyl radicals are 0.43×10^{-11} cm^3/molecule per second at 19 °C [32], and 0.53×10^{-11} cm^3/molecule per second at 23 °C [141]. Atmospheric residence times of 2.7 and 2.2 days, respectively, can be calculated on the basis of these rate constants [44]. These short lifetimes will prevent migration of the chemical to the stratosphere.

The initial reaction product of 1-propanol with a hydroxyl radical is an α-hydroxypropyl. By analogy with the irradiation of ethanol in an NO_x-air atmosphere, these radicals are expected to react with oxygen, almost exclusively with hydrogen abstraction from the hydroxyl group to produce propionaldehyde [34].

Hydrolysis or light-induced degradation of 1-propanol in water cannot be expected. No data are available on abiotic degradation in soil.

4.3 Biotransformation

4.3.1 Biodegradation

The results of the determination of the biological oxygen demand (BOD) of 1-propanol in various sources at 20 °C, using dilution methods, are summarized in Table 3. Unless otherwise stated, they are expressed as a percentage of the theoretical oxygen demand (ThOD), which is 2.40 g oxygen/g 1-propanol. The chemical oxygen demand (COD) was reported to be 91% of the ThOD [149].

Gerhold & Malaney [66] added 1-propanol to undiluted activated sludge and found an oxygen uptake of 37% of the ThOD in 24 h.

There are two reports on anaerobic biodegradation. Typical 1-propanol removal efficiencies for an anaerobic lagoon treatment facility with a retention time of 15 days were 77% and 81% after loading with concentrated wastes [92]. In closed bottle studies, 1-propanol was completely degraded anaerobically by an acetate-enriched culture, derived from a seed of domestic sludge. The culture started to utilize cross-fed, 1-propanol after 4 days, at a rate of 110 mg/litre per day. In a mixed reactor with a 20-day retention time, seeded by the same culture, 41% removal was achieved in the 20 days following 70 days of acclimation to give a final 1-propanol concentration of 10 000 mg/litre [38].

Table 3. BOD of 1-propanol

Dilution water	Source or seed material	Adaptation (+/−)	BODx[a]	Value (% ThOD)	Reference
Fresh	domestic waste water		BOD$_5$ BOD$_{20}$	64 75	[149]
	domestic waste water		BOD$_5$	93	[202]
	synthetic waste water		BOD$_5$	97	[202]
	activated sludge	+	BOD$_5$	99 b	[144]
Salt	domestic waste water	−	BOD$_5$ BOD$_{20}$	43 73	[149]

[a] BOD$_x$ = biological oxygen demand after x days of incubation.
[b] Expressed as percentage of the COD.

4.3.2 Bioaccumulation

1-Propanol is completely miscible with water. Its log *n*-octanol/ water partition coefficient is 0.34 [80]. A bioconcentration factor of 0.7 can be calculated using the formula of Veith & Kosian [197]. In addition, the compound is biodegradable. In view of these data, no bioaccumulation is expected.

5. ENVIRONMENTAL LEVELS AND HUMAN EXPOSURE

5.1 Environmental Levels

The rapid chemical and physical removal of 1-propanol from air and water is reflected in the few reports indicating its presence in these compartments. No data are available on the occurrence of the compound in soil.

In 11 samples of air from a city in the USA in 1982, the average concentration of 1-propanol was 0.00005 mg/m^3, while the compound was not detected in 18 rural samples [174].

1-Propanol at a concentration of 73 mg/m^3 was detected in the air beneath the surface of 1 out of 6 landfill sites sampled in the United Kingdom. This particular site was used for the disposal of domestic waste [216]. 1-Propanol was also detected in the leachate from two sanitary land-fill sites in the USA. This would, at least partly, have originated from the anaerobic degradation of organic compounds by microorganisms [30, 102]. 1-Propanol was identified as a product of the bacterial fermentation of dead blue-green algae [214], fish spoilage bacteria [3], and *Kluyveromyces lactis* yeast [78]. The compound was measured in fresh swine manure [215].

5.2 General Population Exposure

1-Propanol was detected in drinking-water samples in the USA at a concentration of 0.001 mg/litre [165].

Alcoholic beverages nearly always contain 1-propanol as a product of fermentation. Beer contains up to 195 mg/litre [17], wine up to 116 mg/litre [18], various types of spirit up to 3520 mg/litre [130], and neat ethanol up to 2910 mg/litre [9, 19, 146, 140, 186, 148].

Studies summarized in Table 4 show the presence of low levels of 1-propanol as a flavour volatile in a variety of foodstuffs and non-alcoholic drinks. According to Stofberg & Grundschober [179], most of the 1-propanol that they found in the foodstuffs and drinks was of natural origin, not added.

30

Table 4. 1-Propanol as a flavour volatile in foodstuffs and non-alcoholic drinks[a]

Foodstuff/drink		Reference
Common name	Scientific name	
Kefir culture		[142]
Cream culture		[142]
Filberts (roasted)	*Corylus avellana*	[103]
Raw milk		[97]
Heat-treated milk		[97]
Kumazasa Sasa albo-marginata		[134]
Heated triolein [b]		[123]
Boiled buckwheat flour	*Fagopyrum esculentum*	[211]
Ripe tomato, tomato juice, puree, and paste	*Lycopersicon esculentum*	[39]
Kogyoku apple		[212]
Apple and apple juice		[179]
Tomato	*Lycopersicon esculentum*	[179]
White bread		[179]
Butter		[179]
Cheddar/Swiss cheese		[179]
Swiss Gruyere cheese		[22]
Soy sauce (Shoyu)		[135]
Fish sauce (Patis)		[163]
Pigweed	*Amaranthus retroflexus*	[58]
Winged bean (raw/roasted)	*Psophocarpus tetragonalobus*	[47]
Soybean (raw, roasted)	*Glycine max*	[47]
Potato tuber	*Solanum tuberosum*	[205, 206]
Roasted watermelon seeds	*Citrullus colocynthis*	[175]
Babaco fruit	*Carica pentagona*	[168]
Tilsit cheese		[133]
Endive	*Cichorium endivia*	[73]
Valancia orange juice		[127]

[a] Detected by GC/FI, GC/FP, or GC/MS.
[b] The triolein was heated at 185 °C with periodic injection of steam, during 75 h.

5.3 Occupational Exposure

Workers are potentially exposed to 1-propanol during the production of the compound itself or its derivatives, or during its use in solvent-type applications. No data are available on levels of exposure.

6. KINETICS AND METABOLISM

6.1 Absorption

6.1.1 Animals

Data on absorption following inhalation or dermal exposure are not available.

Oral exposure of Wistar rats to one dose of 3004 mg 1-propanol/kg body weight in water resulted in a maximum blood concentration of 1860 mg 1-propanol/litre, 1.5 h after exposure [11].

In rabbits receiving single intraperitoneal doses of 800, 1200, or 1600 mg 1-propanol/kg body weight in saline, maximum blood concentrations, attained within 0.5 h, were proportional to the dose [139].

Blood levels of 1-propanol were determined in groups of 3 adult [200–300g) Sprague-Dawley rats following 1,10, or 19 consecutive 7-h daily exposures to measured concentrations of 9001 or 14 893 mg/m^3 (3659 or 6054 ppm), and after a single exposure to 23 968 mg/m^3 (9743 ppm). Immature (110–120 g) females of the same strain were also evaluated following a single 7-h exposure to 23 968 mg/m^3 (9743 ppm). In the immature females, the blood level of 1-propanol was 1640 mg/litre. The blood levels in adult rats following a single exposure were 26 mg/litre (9001 mg/m^3), 42 mg/litre (14 893 mg/m^3), and 66 mg/litre (23 968 mg/m^3). Blood levels in adults were not detected following 10 and 19 exposures to 9001 mg/m^3 (3659 ppm), and were 49 and 43 mg/litre after exposure to 14 893 mg/m^3 (6054 ppm) [132].

6.1.2 Human beings

Ten human volunteers drank 1-propanol in ethanolic orange juice at doses of 3.75 mg 1-propanol and 1200 mg ethanol/kg body weight over a period of 2 h. At the end of this period, the average peak blood concentration of 1-propanol was 0.85 ± 0.17 mg/litre (mean ± standard deviation). When the blood samples taken at comparable times were analysed after incubation with aryl sulfatase

32

(EC 3.1.6.1), an average peak concentration of 0.92 ± 0.19 mg/litre was measured, just after exposure [19]. These data suggest that 1-propanol is not extensively sulfate conjugated.

6.2 Distribution

i.2.1 Animals

1-Propanol, a compound that is infinitely soluble in water, is rapidly distributed throughout the body of various species [1, 157]. When ^{14}C-1-propanol was administered intraperitoneally to rats in a single dose of 450 mg/kg body weight, the concentrations of 1-propanol and/or its metabolites in the blood, liver, and brain were similar 5 min after administration. Radioactivity was detected in the nuclear and mitochondrial fractions of liver and brain homogenates. Maximum levels were reached later in these subcellular fractions than in the whole organs [125].

i.2.2 Human beings

In the presence of other aliphatic alcohols, after oral ingestion of an alcoholic beverage, 1-propanol appears to be widely distributed throughout the human body [14, 15].

1-Propanol was shown *in vitro* to bind to human α-fetoprotein with a higher affinity than either methanol or ethanol, which is in accordance with its higher hydrophobicity [87].

6.3 Metabolic Transformation

i.3.1 Animals

The metabolic fate of 1-propanol is shown in Fig. 1. 1-Propanol is primarily oxidized to propionaldehyde by the non-specific cytosolic enzyme alcohol dehydrogenase (ADH) (EC 1.1.1.1) followed by conversion to propionic acid [139]. ADH activity is known to be the rate-limiting factor in the elimination of aliphatic alcohols. The Michaelis-Menten constant (K_m) of ADH purified from rat, dog,

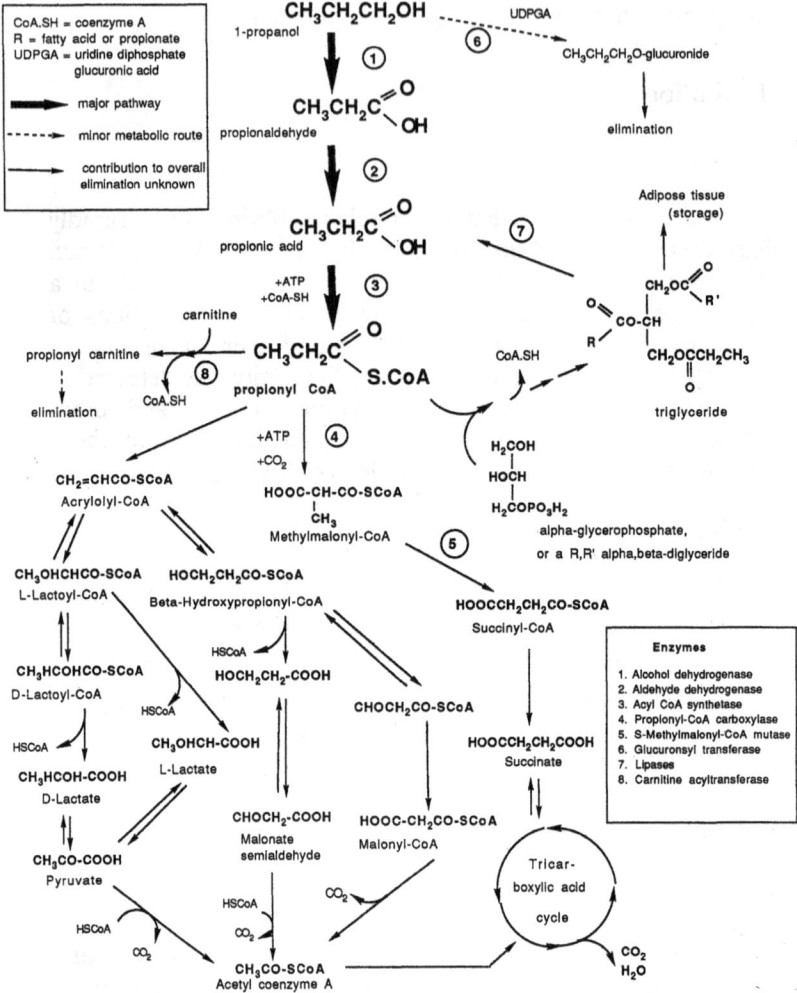

Fig. 1. Proposed metabolic fate of 1-propanol in mammals.

horse, or human liver with 1-propanol as substrate, is lower than the K_m for ethanol or 2-propanol [45, 7, 72]. Hence, 1-propanol is a better substrate for ADH than ethanol or 2-propanol and retards the elimination of the latter compounds. It has been shown *in vitro* that rat and rabbit liver microsomal oxidases (EC 1.14.14.1) are also capable of oxidizing 1-propanol to propionaldehyde [188, 126]. The relative affinity of the microsomal ethanol oxidizing system (MEOS) for 1-propanol is about three times higher than for ethanol and is in accordance with their relative hydrophobicities. In rabbits, cytochrome P-450 isozyme 3a is responsible for the microsomal metabolism of alcohols [126], in rats, it is isozyme P-450j, and in human liver, isozyme P-450 HLj [160]. These forms of cytochrome P-450 are inducible by ethanol [126, 160], it may therefore be expected that in individuals who regularly consume ethanol, the MEOS will contribute to the overall oxidation of 1-propanol. The metabolism of N-nitrosodimethylamine and 1-propanol is mediated by the same isozyme of cytochrome P-450 [160]. Tomera et al., [191] showed that 1-propanol inhibited the metabolism of N-nitrodimethylamine in isolated perfused rat livers .

As in the case of propionic acid formed from the catabolism of odd chain fatty acids, propionic acid arising from the oxidation of 1-propanol can form a coenzyme A (CoA) conjugate [157] catalysed by acyl CoA synthetase (EC 6.2.1.3). A number of different pathways for the further metabolism of propionyl-CoA (Fig. 1) are discussed. However, the relative contribution of each of these to the overall elimination of 1-propanol is not known.

(i) In the methylmalonyl pathway, propionyl-CoA is carboxylated to methylmalonyl-CoA, this is followed by trans-carboxylation to succinyl-CoA, which subsequently enters the tricarboxcylic acid cycle to be metabolized to carbon dioxide and water.

(ii) In the lactate pathway, the propionyl-CoA is dehydrogentated to acrylolyl-CoA, α-hydration gives L-lactoyl-CoA, which is hydrolysed to lactate.

(iii) In another pathway the acrylolyl-CoA is hydrated to 3-hydroxy-propionyl-CoA, deacylation and oxidation result in the formation of malonic acid semialdehyde, which is converted to acetyl-CoA. These reactions, which constitute the major pathways for propionic acid metabolism in plant mitochondria, also occur in animals.

(iv) The propionyl CoA may also participate in triglyceride synthesis.

(v) The obligatory formation of propionyl carnitine required for the transport of propionic acid into mitochrondria may also be an excretory pathway under conditions of high carnitine and propionic acid concentrations [158, 153].

Propionic acid and/or propionyl-CoA are potent inhibitors of several mitochondrial enzymes required for fatty acid oxidation, gluconeogenesis, and ureagenesis; their inhibitory effects can be reversed with carnitine [24, 23]. The formation of propionyl-CoA, its metabolism and effects on oxidative metabolism provide an explanation for the hepatic effects observed in rats after high oral exposure to 1-propanol (section 8.2) and for the biochemical effects seen in some studies (section 8.3.1). Indeed the accumulation of acyl-CoA esters, including propionyl-CoA, is implicated in the pathogenesis of Reye syndrome [43].

6.4 Elimination and Excretion

Aliphatic alcohols may be eliminated from the body via expired air or the urine. Theoretically, urinary metabolites may arise from oxidation or from conjugation with glucuronic acid or sulfate. There are no reports of the excretion of unchanged 1-propanol in expired air or urine and, following an oral dose to rabbits of 800 mg/kg, only 0.9% was found in the urine as propyl-glucuronide and none as a sulfate conjugate [100].

6.4.1 Animals

Available *in vivo* data, reviewed by Rietbrock & Abshagen [157], showed that the elimination of 1-propanol was dose independent above a single oral dose of 1000 mg/kg body weight in rats and above a single intraperitoneal dose of 1200 mg/kg body weight in rabbits [139, 1, 11]. The rate of the zero-order elimination of the compound from the blood of rats that had received a single oral dose of 3000 mg/kg body weight was found to be 510 mg/kg body weight per hour [11]. At lower doses, the elimination rate was first order. When rats were given a single oral dose of 1000 mg/kg body weight, the half-life of 1-propanol was 45 min [1]. The overall metabolism and elimination of 1-propanol are described in section 6.3.1. In mice, a half-life of 57 min was estimated for the exponential elimination phase following a single oral exposure [1]. This should be considered an approximation because there were only 2 or 3 time points per dose.

In vitro, the elimination of 1-propanol from the perfusate of rat liver was also shown to be saturable, a zero-order phase being succeeded below a concentration of 78 mg/litre by an exponential phase with a half-life of 14 min [7].

6.4.2 Human beings

No data were available describing the elimination kinetics of 1-propanol in human beings.

When 10 volunteers drank 1-propanol in ethanolic orange juice at doses of 3.75 mg 1-propanol and 1200 mg ethanol/kg body weight over a period of 2 h, the compound was detected in the blood and in the urine, partly as glucuronide. The total urinary excretion of 1-propanol was 2.1% of the dose. The urinary levels of 1-propanol were lower when the amount of simultaneously ingested ethanol was less, showing competition for ADH between 1-propanol and the ethanol overdose [19, 20].

7. EFFECTS ON ORGANISMS IN THE ENVIRONMENT

7.1 Aquatic Organisms

A summary of acute aquatic toxicity data is presented in Table 5. In none of these studies was the concentration of 1-propanol reported to have been measured. In view of the volatility of the compound, it can be expected that the toxic effects observed in the open-system studies occurred at lower concentrations than the nominal ones.

Several short-term studies have also been conducted. Seiler et al. [167] determined the breakpoint of bioinhibition for a total of 20 strains of several bacterial groups prevalent in a waste-water treatment plant in the chemical industry, i.e., *Zoogloea, Alcaligenes,* and *Pseudomonas*. After one week of static exposure to 1-propanol in an open system at 30 °C, 100% growth inhibition occurred at concentrations of 10 000–30 000 mg/litre of medium. No analysis for the compound was reported.

Inhibition of cell multiplication of blue algae (*Microcystis aeruginosa*) and green algae (*Scenedesmus quadricauda*) reached 100% after 8 days of static exposure to 255 and 3100 mg 1-propanol/litre water, respectively, in a closed system at 27 °C and a pH of 7 [25, 27].

7.2 Terrestrial Organisms

7.2.1 Insects

The toxicity of 1-propanol for insect larvae is summarized in Table 5. In static tests, the 48-h LC_{50} values for adults of the fruit fly strains of *Drosophila melanogaster* and *Drosophila simulans* were between 18 490 and 24 120 mg/litre of nutrient medium and 11 260 and 12 860 mg/litre of nutrient medium, respectively [46].

38

Table 5. Acute aquatic toxicity of 1-propanol

Organism	Temperature (°C)	pH	Dissolved oxygen (mg/litre)	Hardness (mg/CaCO$_3$/litre)	System[a]	Exposure period	Parameter	Nominal concentration (mg/litre)	Reference
FRESHWATER									
Bacteria									
Pseudomonas putida	25	7			closed	16 h	TT[b]	2 700	[27]
Microorganisms									
Activated sludge	21	7.4–8			closed	3 h	50% inhibition of respiration	1 000	[105]
Acclimated mixed waste-water culture	30	6.8			closed	1.2 h	50% inhibition of respiration	19 085	[196]
Protozoa									
Entosiphon sulcatum	25	6.9			closed	72 h	TT[b]	38	[26]
Chilomonas paramecium	20	6.9			closed	48 h	TT[b]	175	[29]
Uronema parduczi	25	6.9			closed	20 h	TT[b]	568	[28]
Algae									
Selenastrum capricornutum	25–26				closed	96 h	NOAEC[c]	2 000	[172]
Scenedesmus pannonicus	25–26				closed	48 h	NOAEC[c]	2 900	[172]
Chlorella pyrenoidosa	25–26				closed	48 h	NOAEC[c]	1 150	[172]

Table 5 (contd).

Organism	Temperature (°C)	pH	Dissolved oxygen (mg/litre)	Hardness (mg/CaCO$_3$/litre)	System[a]	Exposure period	Parameter	Nominal concentration (mg/litre)	Reference
Coelenterate									
Hydra oligactis	17	8.2–8.4	≥ 5		closed	48 h	LC$_{50}$	6 800	[170]
Worms									
Flatworm (*Dugesia*)	20	8.2–8.4	≥ 5		closed	48 h	LC$_{50}$	4 700	[170]
Tubificid worm	20	8.2–8.4	≥ 5		closed	48 h	LC$_{50}$	9 200	[170]
Molluscs									
Giant pond snail (*Lymnea stagnalis*)	20	8.2–8.4	≥ 5		closed	48 h	LC$_{50}$	6 500	[170]
Crustaceans									
Water flea (*Daphnia magna*)[e]	20	8	≥ 2	250	open	24 h	EC$_{50}$[d] EC$_0$ EC$_{100}$	4 415 3 336 5 909	[27]
Water flea (*Daphnia pulex*)[e]	19 19				open open	48 h 48 h	LC$_{50}$ LC$_{50}$	7 080 3 025	[33] [33]
Water flea (*Daphnia cucullata*)[e]	19				open	48 h	LC$_{50}$	5 820	[33]

Table 5 (contd).

Isopod (Asellus aquaticus)	20	8.2–8.4	≥5	209	closed	48 h	LC_{50}	2 500	[170]
Scud (Gammarus pulex)	20	8.2–8.4	≥5	209	closed	48 h	LC_{50}	1 000	[170]
Insects									
Mosquito larvae (Aedes aegypti)	22–24				open	4 h	LC_{50}	10 450	[107]
Mosquito larvae (Aedes aegypti, Culex pipiens)	26	8.2–8.4	≥5	209	open	48 h	LC_{50} LC_{0}	4 400, 4 800 3 200, 3 600	[172]
Midge larvae (Chironomus gr. thummi)	20	8.2–8.4	≥5	209	closed	48 h	LC_{50}	2 350	[170]
Leech larvae (Erpobdella octoculata)	20	8.2–8.4	≥5	209	closed	48 h	LC_{50}	1 400	[170]
Dragon fly larvae (Ischnura elegans)	20	8.2–8.4	≥5	209	closed	48 h	LC_{50}	4 200	[170]
Stonefly larvae (Nemoura cinerea)	20	8.2–8.4	≥5	209	closed	48 h	LC_{50}	1 520	[170]
Mayfly larvae (Cloeon dipterum)	20	8.2–8.4	≥5	209	closed	48 h	LC_{50}	3 110	[170]
Corixa punctata (larvae)	20	8.2–8.4	≥5	209	closed	48 h	LC_{50}	2 000	[170]
Fish									
Creek chub (Semotilus atromaculatus)	15–21	8.3		98	open	24 h	LC_{0}	200	[68]
Golden orfe (Leuciscus idus melanotus)	20	7–8	≥5	200–300	closed	48 h	LC_{50} LC_{0}	4 320, 4 560 3 600, 4 000	[99]

41

Table 5 (contd).

Organism	Temperature (°C)	pH	Dissolved oxygen (mg/litre)	Hardness (mg/CaCO$_3$/litre)	System[a]	Exposure period	Parameter	Nominal concentration (mg/litre)	Reference
Fathead minnow (Pimephales promelas)	20	8.2–8.4	≥5	209	open	48 h	LC$_{50}$ LC$_0$	5 000 2 600	[172]
Rainbow trout (Salmo gairdneri)	15	7–8	≥5	98	open	48 h	LC$_{50}$ LC$_0$	3 200 2 000	[172]
Paddy fish (Oryzias latipes)	24	8.2–8.4	≥5	209	open	48 h	LC$_{50}$ LC$_0$	5 900 4 400	[172]
Amphibia									
South African clawed toad (Xenopus laevis)	20	8.2–8.4	≥5	209	open	48 h	LC$_{50}$	4 000	[171]
Mexican axolotl (Ambystoma mexicanum)	20	8.2–8.4	≥5	209	open	48 h	LC$_{50}$	4 000	[171]
SEA WATER									
Bacteria									
Photobacterium phosphorerum	15				closed	15 min	50% light reduction	8 686	[84]
	5				closed	5 min 15 min	50% light reduction	17 700 18 400	[48]

42

Table 5 (contd).

Crustacea

Brine shrimp (Artemia salina)	24		open	24 h	LC$_{50}$	4 200	[149]f
Harpacticoid copepod (Nitocra spinipes)	21	7.9	≥ 5	96 h	LC$_{50}$	2 300	[12]g

Fish

Bleak (Alburnus alburnus)	10	7.9	≥ 5	open	96 h	LC$_{50}$	3 800	[12]g

a Static systems used in all experiments reported.
b TT = toxic threshold for inhibition of cell multiplication.
c NOAEC = no-observed-adverse-effect-concentration; effect is growth inhibition.
d Effect is complete immobilization.
e Age of Daphnia was 24 h for Daphnia magna and Daphnia pulex, and 11 ± 1 day for Daphnia cucullata.
f Salinity was 2.8%.
g Salinity was 0.7%.

7.2.2 Plants

The effects of 1-propanol on the rate of seed germination have been investigated on several occasions. Total inhibition of the germination of barley grains was reached after incubation for 4 days at 18 °C on filter papers absorbing a solution containing 8050 mg 1-propanol/litre water [40]. The germination of white amaranth (*Amaranthus albus*) seeds was stimulated in a dose-related manner after 5 h incubation at 25 °C on filter papers moistened with a solution containing 3600–36 050 mg 1-propanol/litre water [36]. Reynolds [36] measured 50% inhibition of germination of lettuce (*Lactuca sativa*) seeds after incubation for 3 days at 30 °C on agar containing 3065 mg 1-propanol/litre. The percentage germination and the axis length of soya bean (*Glycine max*) seeds, with the testa removed, were not reduced after exposure to pure 1-propanol for 2 h. After treatment with a 50% (v/v) 1-propanol/water mixture for 2 min, germination was almost completely inhibited and axis length was reduced [150].

1-Propanol was marginally effective in breaking the dormancy of seeds of genetically pure dormant lines of wild oat (*Avena fatua*) after 5 days of exposure to solutions containing up to 1202 mg/litre. Seed viability was affected at higher concentrations [2].

When excised seedling roots of maize (*Zea mays*) were treated by vacuum infiltration in a 5% solution of 1-propanol in water, 3 times for 60 seconds, and then incubated anaerobically at 28 °C, nitrite accumulation increased by 10 times or more, the utilization of nitrate increased, and the utilization of exogenous nitrite was inhibited. These effects were enhanced under aerobic conditions [75]. Dry et al. [51] observed that stimulation of nitrite accumulation in pea and wheat roots under aerobic conditions was accompanied by a decline in the cellular levels of glucose-6-phosphate. It was suggested by Gray & Cresswell [75] that an increase in the utilization of nitrate was related to increased access of nitrate to the site of nitrate metabolism as a result of an increase in membrane permeability.

44

8. EFFECTS ON EXPERIMENTAL ANIMALS AND *IN VITRO* TEST SYSTEMS

8.1 Single Exposures

8.1.1 Mortality

The available LD_{50}s for various animal species are summarized in Table 6. Based on mortality estimates, 1-propanol exhibits low toxicity, except in very young rats. Oral LD_{50} values for several animal species range between 1870 and 6800 mg/kg body weight. For very young rats, oral LD_{50}s of 560–660 mg/kg body weight have been reported [152].

An intraperitoneal dose of 785 mg 1-propanol/kg was lethal to 10 out of 10 C57B/6J and 10 out of 10 DBa/2J mice, but a dose of 392 mg/kg did not cause any deaths in either strain [183]. An LD_{16} of 450 mg/kg was reported in rats after intraperitoneal administration.

When rats were exposed to 1-propanol vapour for 4 h at a concentration of approximately 9840 mg/m^3, 2 out of 6 died within 14 days [173].

8.1.2 Signs of intoxication

Osborne-Mendel or Sherman rats of both sexes receiving a lethal oral dose of undiluted 1-propanol became comatose within a few minutes [187]. Deep narcosis occurred in mice exposed through inhalation of 1-propanol at a concentration of 50 mg/litre for 2 h.

Very young rats (60–100 g) of an unspecified strain and of both sexes, received a single oral dose of between 150 and 3000 mg undiluted 1-propanol/kg body weight. Animals that died showed hyperaemia, vacuolation, and dilated sinusoids in the liver, and hyperaemia, tubular cloudy swelling, and tubular necrosis in the kidneys [152].

When anaesthetized Sprague-Dawley rats were made to inspire 160 mg of the undiluted compound, all 9 exposed rats died within

Table 6. LD$_{50}$s for 1-propanol

Species	Sex	Route of exposure	Observation period	LD$_{50}$ (mg/kg body weight)	Comments	Reference
Wistar rat (non-fasted)	male	oral	14 days	1870	vehicle: wate	[173]
Osborne-Mendel or Sherman rat	male, female	oral	until recovery	6500	undiluted	[187]
CD mouse	not reported	oral	3 days	6800	undiluted	[164]
Rabbit	male, female	oral	1 day	2820		[130]
Wistar rat	male	intravenous	5 days	590	vehicle: water	[190]
H mouse	male, female	intravenous, intravenous	5 days, not reported	697, 1090	vehicle: water, vehicle: water	[190], [40]
Chinchilla rabbit	male, female	intravenous	5 days	483	vehicle: water	[190]
Wistar rat	male	intraperitoneal	5 days	2247	vehicle: water	[190]
H mouse	male	intraperitoneal	5 days	3695	vehicle: water	[190]
Syrian hamster	male	intraperitoneal	5 days	2337	vehicle: water	[190]
Guinea-pig		intraperitoneal	5 days	1208	vehicle: water	[190]
New Zealand rabbit	male	dermal	14 days	4050	1/10 of body surface exposed under cover for 24 h	[173]

165 min, 6 of them dying immediately from respiratory arrest. All controls survived and were killed 24 h later. It was not reported whether the latter were sham-exposed or not. The average absolute lung weight of the exposed rats was increased by 92%. The lungs showed oedema and small areas of focal haemorrhage [65].

Special studies on neurotoxic and behavioural effects, and on biochemical effects are described in sections 8.3 and 8.4.

8.1.3 *Skin, eye, and respiratory tract irritation; sensitization*

Data for skin and eye irritation were not available. One skin sensitization test has been reported concerning an ear-swelling test on CF1 mice. No sensitization was observed [61]. Although the test requires further validation, it correctly discriminated between a number of known positive and negative human sensitizing agents. The authors claim it to be an accurate, sensitive, and efficient method for evaluating delayed contact sensitization.

The sensory irritation of 1-propanol was investigated using a 50% reflex decrease in the respiratory rate of mice (RD_{50}) as an index. Only the heads of the mice were exposed. An exposure-related effect was found with RD_{50} values for the first 10 min of exposure of 31 252 mg/m^3 for Swiss Webster mice [101] and 33 604 mg/m^3 for CF-1 mice [108]. The potential of 1-propanol as a respiratory irritant is therefore low.

8.2 Repeated Exposures

Only a few data are available concerning the oral exposure of animals.

When 3 male and 3 female rats of unspecified strain were exposed to 4 daily oral doses of 2160 mg undiluted 1-propanol, no deaths occurred and no gross pathological signs were seen in the liver [187].

In a group of 6 male rats of unspecified strain, receiving drinking-water containing 1-propanol at a concentration of 60 090 mg/litre for 4 months, food consumption, body weight gain, and liver histopathology were comparable to those of the control group. It should be noted that the authors reported a dose rate of 3 mg/kg body weight per day, while a dose rate of approximately 3000 mg/kg body weight per day seems more appropriate, assuming a water consumption of 20 ml/day and a body weight of 400 g [85].

Groups of 10 Wistar rats were exposed to 1-propanol in the drinking-water at a concentration of 320 000 mg/litre (calculated by the Task Group to be equivalent to approximately 16 000 mg/kg body weight per day, on the basis of the assumptions made above) for 5, 9, or 13 weeks. Control groups comprised 10 rats each. The exposed rats gradually became weak, losing their appetites and showing a decreased body weight gain. Electron microscopic studies of the liver showed irregularly shaped megamitochondria with few cristae, and normally sized but irregularly shaped mitochondria with a decreased number of cristae. Biochemical changes included a decreased state 3 respiration using glutamate as a substrate and decreased specific activities of cytochrome c oxidase (EC 1.9.3.1) and monoamine oxidase (EC 1.4.3.4) [203].

8.3 Neurotoxic and Behavioural Effects

In one study on anaesthetized mongrel dogs, it was shown that 1-propanol, as well as other primary alcohols, could increase the permeability of the blood–brain barrier. The dogs received a sodium fluorescein solution and 0.578 mg 1-propanol in saline, intravenously. The concentration of sodium fluorescein in the cerebrospinal fluid rose to a maximum within 10 min and returned to control levels, 3 h after exposure [78].

The oral ED_{50} (1440 mg/kg body weight) for narcosis in rabbits exposed to 1-propanol was 4 times lower than that for ethanol [129]. Deep narcosis occurred in mice exposed through inhalation to 50 mg 1-propanol/litre for 2 h, and a 40-min exposure to 2.3 mg/litre reduced the unconditioned flexor response in rabbits. When rabbits were intravenously infused with 1-propanol at a rate of 9–30 mg/min per kg body weight, positional nystagmus with an inhibited rotatory response was observed at and above a blood concentration of 900 mg/litre [137].

The intraperitoneal ED_{50} for loss of righting reflex in Swiss Webster mice administered 1478 mg 1-propanol/kg body weight was 2.8 times lower than that for ethanol [117]. When C57BL/6J or DBA/2J mice were given a single dose of 1-propanol intraperitoneally, both strains showed decreased activity in the open field test at 392 mg/kg body weight, but the decrease was not significant. All mice given 785 and 1570 mg/kg body weight died [183]. The rotarod performance of Swiss-Cox mice decreased in a dose-related manner after single oral doses of 1-propanol of 2000 or 4000 mg/kg body weight. A dose of 1000 mg/kg body weight did not cause behavioural impairment. When the study was repeated on days 4, 6, 7, and 8 after the first trial, tolerance did not develop [1].

The threshold for the induction of ataxia in Sprague-Dawley rats following intraperitoneal exposure was 799 mg/kg body weight [119]. In a tilted plane test, the performance of rats decreased by an average of 71% after oral exposure to 2000 mg/kg body weight. On a molar basis, 1-propanol was 2.5 times as intoxicating as ethanol [204].

According to several investigators, depression of the central nervous system by 1-propanol was related to interactions with neuronal membranes. Lyon et al. [117] observed a high correlation between the narcotic potencies of the aliphatic alcohols, including 1-propanol, in mice and their ability to disorder the brain synaptosomal plasma membrane *in vitro*, as measured by electron paramagnetic resonance, which was in turn related to membrane solubility. A change in membrane fluidity was shown to occur in isolated synaptosomal plasma membranes of rat cortex *in vitro* by a decrease in 1,6-diphenyl-1,3,5-hexatriene fluorescence polarization [81].

Functional loss due to disruption of membrane integrity by 1-propanol was observed *in vitro*. The action potentials of the sciatic nerves of the toad (*Bufo marinus*) [155] and of giant axons of the squid (*Loligo forbesi*) [143] were decreased by 1-propanol. In isolated rat phrenic nerve-diaphragm, 1-propanol increased the amplitudes of end-plate and miniature end-plate potentials and the number of quanta of acetylcholine of end-plate potentials [62]. The compound also affected the rate of decay of postsynaptic currents in the neuromuscular junction of the crayfish (*Cherax destructor*) [200], and in the phrenic nerve-diaphragm of the rat [62].

Effects on the ionic currents underlying the changes in excitability described above were also investigated *in vitro*. 1-Propanol

4

inhibited both the K^+-stimulated and the Na^+-dependent influx of Ca^{2+} ions into isolated rat brain synaptosomes [80, 81, 124], and the influx of Na^+ ions into rat brain synaptosomes [128]. It decreased the Na^+ and K^+ currents in the giant axons of the squid (*Loligo forbesi*) [143], and in sciatic nerve fibres of the clawed toad (*Xenopus laevis*) [6]. The interference of 1-propanol with the transport of Ca^{2+} ions across biological membranes was also shown *in vitro* by the inhibition of Ca^{2+} ion-induced contractions of guinea-pig ileum [213], and *in vivo*, in rats, by a decrease in regional brain Ca^{2+} ion levels, 30 min after one intraperitoneal dose of 2000 mg/kg body weight [159].

The disruption of neuronal membranes by 1-propanol was also thought to explain its inhibitory action on the binding of dihydromorphine to isolated mouse brain caudate membranes [185] and on membrane-bound guanylate cyclase (EC 4.6.1.2) in intact murine neuroblastoma N1E-115 cells [172]. The activation by 1-propanol of membrane-bound adenylate cyclase (EC 4.6.1.1) from isolated mouse striatal membranes, in the presence of guanine nucleotides, was also suggested to be the result of membrane perturbation [116].

8.4 Biochemical Effects

8.4.1 Effects on lipids in the liver and blood

Oral administration of single doses of 3000 or 6000 mg 1-propanol/kg body weight to Wistar rats caused a transient increase in hepatic triglycerides, which was related to the duration of an elevated blood–1-propanol concentration [10, 11]. Gaillard & Derache [63] did not observe an increase in hepatic triglycerides in Wistar rats, 17 h after a single dose of 6000 mg 1-propanol/kg body weight.

Factors possibly responsible for hepatic triglyceride accumulation include: an increase in hepatic uptake of labelled palmitate [11], an increased esterification of palmitate to form liver triglycerides [10, 11], and decreased palmitate oxidation [11]. The decrease in palmitate oxidation was related to an increase in the hepatic α-hydroxybutyrate/acetoacetate ratio, implying a decrease in the intramitochondrial NAD^+/NADH ratio [11]. An increase in extramitochondrial reducing equivalents, indicated by an increased lactate/pyruvate ratio, was observed *in vitro* by Forsander [60], but not *in vivo* by Beaugé et al. [11].

The effects of 1-propanol on palmitate incorporation into triglycerides appear to depend on the dose, high doses causing inhibition and lower ones leading to an increase. The incorporation of palmitate into serum triglycerides and serum and liver phospholipids, 4.5 h after a single oral dose of 6000 mg 1-propanol/kg body weight to rats, was found to be inhibited, while an increase in hepatic triglyceride accumulation was only observed 8 h after dosing [10]. Three hours after a dose of 3000 mg/kg body weight, the incorporation of palmitate in blood triglycerides was increased concomitantly with an increase in hepatic triglycerides while levels of phospholipids in the liver and blood were unaffected [11]. Similar effects have been noted with ethanol [11].

8.4.2 Effects on microsomal enzymes

The effects of 1-propanol on microsomal enzymes (EC 1.14.14.1) *in vivo* was investigated by Powis [147], who administered a single oral dose of 960 mg/kg body weight to Wistar rats. Twenty four hours after exposure, no effects were observed on the activities of aniline hydroxylase and aminopyrine demethylase in liver microsomes. This study is inadequate to demonstrate an inductive effect of 1-propanol on the microsomal mixed function oxidase system. *In vitro*, 1-propanol inhibited aldrin epoxidase and *p*-aniline hydroxylase in isolated rat liver microsomes via an interaction with cytochrome P-450, which causes a reverse Type I spectral change [41, 210, 189, 161]. At high concentrations, the inhibition of the mixed function monoxygenase system by aliphatic alcohols correlates directly with the lipophilicity of the alcohols, and is probably the result of unspecific effects on the membrane (see section 8.3). The compound did not affect the levels of hepatic microsomal cytochrome P-450, haem, cytochrome b5, and NADPH-cytochrome c reductase (EC 1.6.2.4) in phenobarbital-induced rats [96]. 1-Propanol increased the levels of cytochrome P-450 in cultured chick embryo hepatocytes. The activities of benzphetamine demethylase and UDP-glucuronosyl transferase (EC 2.4.1.17) were also increased [169].

8.4.3 Other biochemical findings

The glutathione level in the liver of Wistar rats administered a single dose of 1660 mg 1-propanol/kg body weight, orally, had decreased by 20%, 6 h after exposure. Lipid peroxidation, as indicated by diene conjugates formation, was increased; ethanol in equivalent doses produced similar effects [199].

The activities of liver ornithine decarboxylase (EC 4.1.1.17) and liver tyrosine aminotransferase (EC 2.6.1.5) increased in partially hepatectomized rats 4 h after one oral dose of 2300 mg 1-propanol/kg body weight or an equivalent dose of ethanol. No effects were observed on levels of alanine aminotransferase (EC 2.6.1.2) in the liver and kidneys, and on levels of ornithine decarboxylase in the kidneys and brain [145].

The effects of 1-propanol on neuronal membrane-bound adenylate cyclase (EC 4.6.1.1) and guanylate cyclase (EC 4.6.1.2) *in vitro* are discussed in section 8.3. 1-Propanol and ethanol, can have different effects on the activity of adenylate cyclase, depending on the concentration of alcohol and the biological system being investigated [178, 192, 93].

When Sprague-Dawley rats inhaled 1-propanol for 6 h at a concentration of 490 mg/m^3, the serum level of testosterone was decreased by 42% immediately after exposure, but not 18 h after exposure. When this exposure regimen was repeated daily over one week, no effects on serum testosterone levels were observed. Serum levels of luteinizing hormone and corticosterone were unchanged at all times [31].

When a crude homogenate of dispersed acinar cells, prepared from guinea-pig pancreas, was incubated with 1-propanol and secretin, the secretin-stimulated activities of adenylate cyclase (EC 4.6.1.1) and cellular cyclic adenosine 3',5'-monophosphate were potentiated at low concentrations of 1-propanol, but the potentiation was reversible. Irreversible inhibition occurred at higher concentrations [192].

8.5 Reproduction, Embryotoxicity, and Teratogenicity

Groups of 15 male Sprague-Dawley rats were exposed to 1-propanol at measured concentrations of 8610 or 15 220 mg/m^3 for 7 h/day over 6 weeks. Beginning on the third day after the last exposure, males were mated for a maximum of 5 days with unexposed females. There was no apparent effect of exposure to 8610 mg/m^3 on mating performance or fertility. After exposure to 15 220 mg/m^3, 17 out of 18 males copulated (as evidenced by the presence of a vaginal plug), but only 2 of 17 mated females became pregnant. The offspring of the exposed males were evaluated postnatally in a battery of behavioural tests. There was no evidence of any exposure-related effect [132].

These investigators also exposed groups of 15 pregnant Sprague-Dawley rats to the same concentrations of 1-propanol on gestation days 1–20. Pregnant females exposed to 15 220 mg/m^3 showed significantly reduced weight gain and food consumption. Their female offspring also showed reduced weight gain up to 3 weeks of age, but there was no consistent effect on male offspring. Litter sizes were not affected. "Several" of the offspring from dams exposed to 15 220 mg/m^3 had crooked tails. Behavioural testing of offspring did not reveal any evidence of an exposure-related effect, though there was an increase in total external, visceral, and skeletal malformations at 23 968 mg/m^3 (9743 ppm) and in total skeletal malformation at 14 893 mg/m^3 (6054 ppm) [132].

The effects of 1-propanol on brain development in the neonatal rat were also studied. A group of 21, 5-day-old Long-Evans rats was exposed to 1-propanol via an artificial milk formula, which was administered through an intragastric catheter for 4 consecutive days. The rats received 12 feeds daily, each lasting 20 min. Doses were 3800, 7500, 3000, or 7800 mg/kg body weight on day 5–8, respectively. Controls received the milk formula only. During the exposure, the exposed pups frequently showed an impaired righting response. After the last exposure, withdrawal symptoms were displayed. Pups were killed at 18 days of age, at which time there was no effect on body weight or on absolute weight of kidneys, heart, or liver. However, the absolute and relative brain weights were decreased in the exposed pups. Biochemical analysis showed that the exposed pups had a decreased amount of DNA in all brain areas examined. Cholesterol levels were decreased in the forebrain and cerebellar samples, while protein levels were decreased only in the forebrain samples [74].

8.6 Mutagenicity

8.6.1 Bacteria

1-Propanol was tested for mutagenic activity using Ame's test without S9; up to 100-μmol/plate was negative with *Salmonella typhimurium* TA-100 [181]. Negative results were also reported in TA 100 and TA-98 with or without metabolic activation, following standard Ame's test protocol [94].

In a reverse mutation assay with *Escherchia coli* CA-274 following a pre-incubation protocol, a 5-fold increase in the number of revertants was observed at a concentration of 4.5% 1-propanol. No metabolic activation system was used [86].

8.6.2 Mammalian cells in vitro

1-Propanol (100 mg/litre once a day for 7 days) did not increase the number of sister chromatid exchanges in Chinese hamster ovary cells [136], or in V79 Chinese hamster lung fibroblasts at 6000 mg/litre for 3 h (with activation) and 28 h (without activation) [200]. It did not increase the number of micronuclei in V79 Chinese hamster lung fibroblasts at 40 200 mg/litre for 1 h [113].

A dose-related increase in the inhibition of metabolic cooperation between hamster V79 cells, a phenomenon believed to reflect carcinogenic promotion ability and not be indicative of genotoxic potential, was observed by Chen et al. [37]. This may be due to the membrane effects of 2-propanol.

8.7 Carcinogenicity

A group of 18 Wistar rats of both sexes received doses of 240 mg 1-propanol/kg body weight, by gavage, twice a week, for their lifetime. Another group of 31 Wistar rats of both sexes received subcutaneous injections of 48 mg compound/kg body weight, twice a week, for their lifetime. Control groups, comprising 25 rats for each route, received saline. It was not reported whether the analytical grade, double-distilled test compound was analysed for the presence of impurities. The average survival time was 570 days for the orally exposed rats, 666 days for the subcutaneously exposed rats, and 643 days for both control groups. The tumour incidence is reported in Table 7. The data were not statistically analysed. It was reported that "nearly all rats" showed liver damage including congestion, steatosis, necrosis, fibrosis, and metaplasia and hyperplasia of the haematopoietic bone marrow parenchyma. However, the incidence of these lesions were not reported [67].

Table 7. Tumour incidence in Wistar rats exposed orally or subcutaneously to 1-propanol for lifetime[a]

Organ/ tissue affected	Tumour type	Incidence			
		oral exposure		sc exposure	
		exposed	controls	exposed	controls
Blood	myeloid leukemia	2/18	0/25	4/31	0/25
Liver	carcinoma	1/18	0/25	0/31	0/25
Liver	sarcoma	2/18	0/25	5/31	0/25
Other	carcinoma	0/18	0/25	3/31[b]	0/25
	sarcoma	0/18	0/25	2/31[c]	0/25
	benign tumours[d]	10/18	3/25	7/31	2/25

[a] From: Gibel et al. [67].
[b] One carcinoma each in kidney, bladder, and uterus.
[c] One sarcoma each in spleen and at injection site.
[d] Mostly papillomas and mammary fibroadenomas.

Although there was an apparent increase in the incidence of liver sarcoma, the study is inadequate for the assessment of carcinogenicity. The dosing schedule did not conform to standard protocol. Too few animals were used in each dose group, the sex ratio of each group was unclear, no data were provided on the histological type of liver sarcoma, no statistical analysis was conducted, the maximum tolerated dose was exceeded, as evidenced by the reported liver damage, and only single dose levels were used. In the case of subcutaneous administration, the exposure route was inappropriate.

9.   EFFECTS ON MAN

9.1 General Population Exposure

9.1.1 Poisoning incidents

One case of poisoning by 1-propanol has been reported. It concerned a 46-year-old woman who was estimated to have consumed approximately half a litre of the compound as a solvent in a cosmetic preparation, probably a hair lotion. It was pointed out that the woman could have ingested this preparation more than once in the past. The woman was found unconscious. She died 4–5 h after ingestion. No other signs or symptoms were reported. Autopsy revealed a "swollen brain" and lung oedema [52].

9.1.2 Controlled human studies

Filter papers moistened with 0.025 ml of a 75% solution of 1-propanol in water were placed on the forearms of a group of 12 volunteers following immersion of the forearms in water at 23 °C for 10 min. The patches were covered for 5 min and then gently blotted. Nine of the 12 persons showed erythema for at least 60 min following exposure. The cutaneous reaction was totally blocked in 4 out of 4 persons after pretreatment with 40% 4-methylpyrazole in hydrophilic ointment 1 h before the challenge, showing, according to the authors, that 1-propanol must be metabolized to propanal before vasoactivity occurs [207].

9.2 Occupational Exposure

A laboratory worker in a company manufacturing hair cosmetics developed allergic reactions in patch tests with chemically pure 1-propanol solutions in water (10–99.5% by volume). This person also reacted to 2-propanol, 1-butanol, 2-butanol, and formaldehyde, but not to ethanol and methanol. Controls were not tested [115].

10. EVALUATION OF HUMAN HEALTH RISKS AND EFFECTS ON THE ENVIRONMENT

10.1 Evaluation of Human Health Risks

10.1.1 Exposure

Exposure of human beings to 1-propanol may occur through ingestion of food and alcoholic beverages containing 1-propanol (e.g., wine and beer 100–200 mg/litre, spirits up to 3500 mg/litre). Inhalation exposure may occur during household use and occupationally during manufacture and processing. Exposure of the general population via inhalation and drinking-water is very low (average concentrations in urban air and drinking-water in the USA, 0.00005 mg/m^3 and drinking-water 0.001 mg/litre, respectively) (section 5).

10.1.2 Health effects

1-Propanol is rapidly absorbed and distributed throughout the body following ingestion. Data on the absorption rate following inhalation are lacking but, in view of the physical properties of the compound, it is also expected to be rapid. Dermal absorption is expected to be slow (section 6).

1-Propanol exhibits low acute toxicity for animals (based on lethality estimates), whether exposed via the dermal, oral, or respiratory route (section 8.1). Exposure to potentially lethal levels may occur in the general population through accidental or intentional ingestion. However, only one case of lethal poisoning by 1-propanol has been reported, which probably reflects its low toxicity and limited use by the public (section 9.1.1). The principal toxic effect of 1-propanol following a single exposure is depression of the central nervous system. Quantitative exposure–effect data on human beings are not available. The most likely acute effects of 1-propanol in man are alcoholic intoxication and narcosis. Animal studies indicate that 1-propanol is 2–4 times as intoxicating as ethanol.

A controlled human study has indicated that 1-propanol may be irritating to hydrated skin. However, the potential of 1-propanol as a respiratory irritant is low (section 8.1.3). Data are inadequate for evaluation of the irritating properties of this compound for the skin, eye, and respiratory tract in human beings, or for evaluation of its sensitizing potential.

The results of limited drinking-water studies on animals suggest that oral exposure to 1-propanol is unlikely to pose a serious health hazard under the usual conditions of human exposure (section 8.2).

Inhalation exposure to a concentration of 15 220 mg/m^3 caused impaired reproductive performance in male rats, but exposure to 8610 mg/m^3 did not. In pregnant rats, 9001 mg/m^3 (3659 ppm) was a NOEL and 14 893 mg/m^3 (6054 ppm) was a LOEL for both maternal and developmental toxicity. Behavioural effects were not detected in offspring whose mothers were exposed during pregnancy to 15 220 mg/m^3, but oral dosing of neonatal rats produced biochemical changes in the brain that were detected 10 days after the last treatment (section 8.5). Inhalation exposure to high concentrations of 1-propanol produced reproductive and developmental toxic effects in male and female rats. These effects occurred in the presence of other overt signs of toxicity in the exposed animals and 1-propanol does not appear to be selectively toxic to male or female reproductive processes. The concentrations required to produce these effects in rats were higher than those likely to be encountered under normal conditions of human exposure.

1-Propanol was negative in assays for point mutations in bacteria. It did not increase the incidence of sister chromatid exchange or micronuclei in mammalian cells *in vitro*. Although these findings suggest that the substance does not have any genotoxic potential, no adequate assessment of mutagenicity can be made on the basis of the limited data available. The results of an *in vitro* test said to predict promotional activity were negative (section 8.6). The available study is inadequate to evaluate the carcinogenicity of 1-propanol in experimental animals (section 8.7). No data are available on the long-term exposure of human populations to 1-propanol. Hence, the carcinogenicity of 1-propanol in human beings cannot be evaluated. Apart from one case of fatal poisoning

59

following ingestion of half a litre of 1-propanol, there are practically no reports on adverse health effects from exposure to 1-propanol either in the general population or in occupational groups (section 9).

The Task Group considers it unlikely that 1-propanol will pose a serious health risk for the general population under normal exposure conditions.

10.2 Evaluation of Effects on the Environment

1-Propanol can be released into the environment during production, processing, storage, transport, use, and waste disposal (section 3). It is transferred from water, soil, and waste-disposal sites to the atmosphere by volatilization, from the atmosphere to water and soil by rain-out, and from soil and waste disposal sites to ground water by leaching. It is difficult to estimate its emission into each compartment. Because of its primary use as a volatile solvent, most of the production volume is eventually released into the atmosphere (section 4.1).

By reacting with hydroxyl radicals and through rain-out, 1-propanol will disappear rapidly from the atmosphere, with a residence time of less than 3 days (section 4.2). Thus, measurable atmospheric levels of 1-propanol are not usually encountered.

Hydrolysis and photolysis are not expected to be important in the removal of 1-propanol from water and soil, but removal occurs rapidly by aerobic and anaerobic biodegradation (section 4.3.1) so that measurable levels are rarely found. Adsorption of 1-propanol on soil particles is poor but it is likely to be mobile in soil and it has been shown to increase the permeability of soil to some aromatic hydrocarbons (section 4.1).

In view of the physical properties of 1-propanol, its potential for bioaccumulation is low (section 4.3.2). Except in the case of accident or inappropriate disposal, 1-propanol does not present a risk for aquatic organisms, insects, or plants at concentrations that usually occur in the environment. However, 1-propanol at concentrations of around 5000 mg/litre in water is lethal to oxygen-using aquatic organisms, indicating that its emission into surface water at this level may result in serious alteration of the local ecosystem (section 7).

11.   RECOMMENDATIONS

1. 1-Propanol has not shown mutagenic potential in the small number of assays performed. A full array of modern genotoxicity tests should be carried out.

2. A single published report suggests carcinogenic activity by 1-propanol, but this study is seriously flawed and cannot be used to evaluate the potential carcinogenicity of 1-propanol. The desirability of a carcinogenesis bioassay of 1-propanol should be considered, on the basis of the outcome of genotoxicity tests.

3. Inhalation exposure to overtly toxic concentrations of 1-propanol produced reproductive and developmental toxicity in experimental animals. In view of the potential for environmental and drinking-water contamination, reproductive and developmental toxicity should be investigated using oral dosing.

4. Epidemiological studies including precise exposure data would assist in an assessment of the occupational hazards from 1-propanol.

5. The unusually uniform level of toxicity in diverse types of aquatic organisms that consume gaseous oxygen, and the exceptionally steep dose–effect curve observed, suggest a nonspecific effect that may not be restricted to 1-propanol. These effects merit investigation.

12. PREVIOUS EVALUATIONS BY INTERNATIONAL BODIES

1-Propanol was considered by the Joint FAO/WHO Expert Committee on Food Additives (JECFA) in its twenty-third report. Specifications were formulated, but no toxicological monograph was prepared, and the substance could not be evaluated on the basis of the data available. Additional toxicological information was available to JECFA at a later meeting, including the results of a limited study in rats suggesting a carcinogenic potential for 1-propanol. In its twenty-fifth report,[a] JECFA noted that life-time feeding studies in rodents were required to resolve the problem of carcinogenicity. A toxicological monograph was prepared. The existing specifications were revised and designated as "tentative", but no ADI was established.

---

[a] WHO Technical Report Series, No. 669, 1981 (*Evaluation of certain food additives*: Twenty-fifth Report of the Joint FAO/WHO Expert Committee on Food Additives).

REFERENCES

1. ABSHAGEN, U. & RIETBROCK, N. (1970) [The mechanism of the 2-propanol oxidation.] *Naunyn-Schmiedebergs Arch. Pharmakol. exp. Pathol.*, **265**: 411-424 (in German).

2. ADKINS, S.W., NAYLOR, J.M., & SIMPSON, G.M. (1984) The physiological basis of seed dormancy in *Avena fatua*.V. Action of ethanol and other organic compounds. *Physiol. Plant.*, **62**: 18-24.

3. AHAMED, A. & MATCHES, J.R. (1983) Alcohol production by fish spoilage bacteria. *J. food Prot.*, **46**: 1055-059.

4. ALLINGER, N.L., CAVA, M.P., DE JONGH, D.C., JOHNSON, C.R., LEBEL, N.A., & STEVENS, C.L. (1971) *Organic chemistry*, New York, Worth Publishers, Inc.

5. ANON. (1984) Propyl alcohol complaint settled by US companies. *Chem. marketing Rep.*, **April 23**: 3, 17.

6. ARHEM, P. & VAN HELDEN, D. (1983) Effects of aliphatic alcohols on myelinated nerve membrane. *Acta physiol. Scand.*, **119**: 105-107.

7. AUTY, R.M. & BRANCH, R.A. (1976) The elimination of ethyl, *n*-propyl, *n*-butyl and isoamyl alcohols by the isolated perfused rat liver. *J. Pharmacol. exp. Ther.*, **197**: 669-674.

8. BALD, E. & MAZURKIEWICZ, B. (1980) Analytical utility of 2-halo-pyridinium salts. Part III. Paper electrophoretic characterization of alcohols as 2-alkoxy-1-methylpyridinium *p*-toluenesulfonates. *Chromatographia*, **13**: 295-297.

9. BEAUD, P. & RAMUZ, A. (1978) Dosage simultané des alcools supérieures, et de l'acetate d'éthyle dans les eaux-de-vie par chromatographie gaz-liquide-solide. *Trav. chim. Aliment. Hyg.*, **69**: 423-430.

10. BEAUGE, F., CLEMENT, M., NORDMANN, J., & NORDMANN, R. (1974) Perturbations du métabolisme hépatique du palmitate [1-^{14}C] déterminée par l'administration de *n*-propanol chez le rat. *Biochimie*, **56**: 1157-1159.

11. BEAUGE, F., CLEMENT, M., NORDMANN, J., & NORDMANN, R. (1979) Comparative effects of ethanol, *n*-propanol and isopropanol on lipid disposal by rat liver. *Chem.-biol. Interact.*, **26**: 155-166.

12. BENGTSSON, B.-E., RENBERG, L., & TARKPEA, M. (1984) Molecular structure and aquatic toxicity: an example with C_1-C_{13} aliphatic alcohols. *Chemosphere*, **13**: 613-622.

13. BILZER, N. & GRUNER, O. (1983) [Critical assessment regarding determination of aliphatic alcohols (congeners in alcoholic drinks) in blood with the aid of head-space analysis.] *Blutalkohol*, 20: 411-421 (in German).

14. BILZER, N. & PENNERS, B.-M. (1985) [Concerning the velocity of reduction and excretion of the attendant substance propanol-1 and isobutanol after drinking whisky of the trade mark Chivas Regal.] *Blutalkohol*, 22: 140-145 (in German).

15. BILZER, N., PENNERS, B.-M., & GRUNER, O. (1985) [Studies about the course of concentration in blood for congener propanol-1 and isobutanol after drinking overseas rum ("Captain Morgan").] *Blutalkohol*, 22: 146-151 (in German).

16. BONTE, W. (1978) [Congener content of wine and similar beverages.] *Blutalkohol*, 15: 392-404 (in German).

17. BONTE, W. (1979) [Congener content of German and foreign beers.] *Blutalkohol*, 16: 108-124 (in German).

18. BONTE, W., DECKER, J., & BUSSE, J. (1978) [Congener content of highproof alcoholic beverages.] *Blutalkohol*, 15: 323-338 (in German).

19. BONTE, W., RUDELL, E., SPRUNG, R., FRAUENRATH, C., BLANKE, E., KUPILAS, G., WOCHNIK, J., & ZAH, G. (1981a) [Experimental investigations concerning the analytical detection of small doses of higher aliphatic alcohols in human blood.] *Blutalkohol*, 18: 399-411 (in German).

20. BONTE, W., SPRUNG, R., RUDELL, E., FRAUENRATH, C., BLANKE, E., KUPILAS, G., WOCHNIK, J., & ZAH, G. (1981b) [Experimental investigations concerning the analytical detection of small doses of higher aliphatic alcohols in human urine.] *Blutalkohol*, 18: 412-426 (in German).

21. BONTE, W., STOPPELMAN, G., RUDELL, E., & SPRUNG, R. (1981c) [Computerized detection of congeners of alcoholic beverages in body fluids.] *Blutalkohol*, 18: 303-310 (in German).

22. BOSSET, J.O. & LIARDON, R. (1984) The aroma composition of Swiss Gruyere cheese. II. The neutral volatile components. *Lebensm.-Wiss. Technol.*, 17: 359-362.

23. BRASS, E.P. & BEYERINCK, R.A. (1987) Interactions of propionate and carnitine metabolism in isolated hepatocytes. *Metabolism*, 36: 781-787.

24. BRASS, E.P., FENNESSEY, P.V. & MILLER, L.V. (1986) Inhibition of oxidative metabolism by propionic acid and its reversal by carnitine in isolated rat hepatocytes. *Biochem. J.*, 236:131-136.

25. BRINGMANN, G. (1975) [Determination of the harmful biological action of water-endangering substances through inhibition of cell multiplication in the blue alga *Microcystis*.] *Ges.-Ing.*, **96**: 238-241 (in German).

26. BRINGMANN, G. (1978) [Determination of the harmful biological action of water-endangering substances on protozoa. I. Bacteria fed flagellates.] *Z. Wasser-Abwasser Forsch.*, 11: 210-215 (in German).

27. BRINGMANN, G. & KUHN, R. (1977) [Limiting values of the harmful action of water-endangering substances on bacteria (*Pseudomonas putida*) and green algae (*Scenedesmus quadricauda*) in the cell multiplication inhibition test.] *Z. Wasser-Abwasser Forsch.*, 10: 87-98 (in German).

28. BRINGMANN, G. & KUHN, R. (1980) [Determination of the harmful biological action of water-endangering substances on protozoa. II. Bacteria fed ciliates.] *Z. Wasser-Abwasser Forsch.*, 13: 26-31 (in German).

29. BRINGMANN, G., KUHN, R., & WINTER, A. (1980) [Determination of the harmful biological action of water-endangering substances on protozoa. III. Saprozoic flagellates.] *Z. Wasser-Abwasser Forsch.*, 13: 170-173 (in German).

30. BURROWS, W.D. & ROWE, R.S. (1975) Ether soluble constituents of landfill leachate. *J. Water Pollut. Control Fed.*, 47: 921-923.

31. CAMERON, A.M., ZAHLSEN, K., HAUG, E., NILSEN, O.G., & EIK-NES, K.B. (1985) Circulating steroids in male rats following inhalation of *n*-alcohols. *Arch. Toxicol.*, Suppl., 8: 422-424.

32. CAMPBELL, I.M., MCLAUGHLIN, D.G., & HANDY, B.J. (1976) Rate constants for reactions of hydroxyl radicals with alcohol vapours at 292 K. *Chem. Phys. Lett.*, **38**: 362-364.

33. CANTON, J.H. & ADEMA, D.M.M. (1978) Reproducibility of short-term and reproduction toxicity experiments with *Daphnia magna* and comparison of the sensitivity of *Daphnia magna* with *Daphnia pulex* and *Daphnia cucullata* in short-term experiments. *Hydrobiologia*, 59: 135-140.

34. CARTER, W.P.L., DARNALL, K.R. GRAHAM, R.A., WINER, A.M., & PITTS, J.N. (1979) Reactions of C_2 and C_4-hydroxy radicals with oxygen. *J. phys. Chem.*, **83**: 2305-2311.

35. CEC (1982) Propan-1-ol chemico-physical data, toxicity data, environmental occurrence, and permissible levels. In: *Report of the Scientific Committee for Food on extraction solvents*, Brussels, Commission of the European Communities, Directorate General for Internal Market and Industrial Affairs, pp. 27-45.

36. CHADOEUF-HANNEL, R. & TAYLORSON, R.B. (1985) Anaesthetic stimulation of *Amaranthus albus* seed germination: interaction with phytochrome. *Physiol. Plant*, 65: 451-454.

37. CHEN, T.-H., KAVANAGH, T.J., CHANG, C.C., & TROSKO, J.E. (1984) Inhibition of metabolic cooperation in Chinese hamster V79 cells by various organic solvents and simple compounds. *Cell Biol. Toxicol.*,1: 155-171.

38. CHOU, W.L.,. SPEECE, R.E., & SIDDIQI, R.H. (1978) Acclimation and degradation of petrochemical wastewater components by methane fermentation. *Biotechnol. Bioeng. Symp.*, 8: 391-414.

39. CHUNG, T.-Y., HAYASE, F., & KATO, H. (1983) Volatile components of ripe tomatoes and their juices, purees and pastes. *Agric. biol. Chem.*, 47: 343-351.

40. CHVAPIL, M., ZAHRADNIK, R., & CMUCHALOVA, B. (1962) Influence of alcohols and potassium salts of xanthogenic acids on various biological objects. *Arch. int. Pharmacodyn. Ther.*, 135: 330-343.

41. COHEN, G.M. & MANNERING, G.J. (1973) Involvement of a hydrophobic site in the inhibition of the microsomal *p*-hydroxylation of aniline by alcohols. *Mol. Pharmacol.*, 9: 383-397.

42. CORBIT, T.E. & ENGEN, T. (1971) Facilitation of olfactory detection. *Perception Psychophysiol.*,10: 433-436.

43. CORKEY, B.E., HALE, D.E., GLENNON, M.C., KELLEY, R.I., COATES, P.M. KILPATRIK, L. & STANLEY, C.A. (1988) Relationship between unusual hepatic acyl coenzyme A profiles and the pathogenesis of Reye syndrome. *J. clin. Invest.* 82: 782-788.

44. CUPITT, L.T. (1980) *Fate of toxic and hazardous materials in the air environment*, Research Triangle Park, North Carolina, Environmental Protection Agency, Environmental Sciences Laboratory, Office of Research and Development (EPA No. 600/3- 80-084, PB 80-221948).

45. DALZIEL, K. & DICKINSON, F.M. (1966) The kinetics and mechanism of liver alcohol dehydrogenase with primary and secondary alcohols as substrates. *Biochem. J.*, 100: 34-46.

46. DAVID, J. & BOCQUET, C. (1976) Compared toxicities of different alcohols for two *Drosophila* sibling species : *D. melanogaster* and *D. simulans. Comp. Biochem. Physiol.*, 54C: 71-74.

47. DEL ROSARIO, R., DE LUMEN, B.O., HABU, T., FLATH, R.A., MON, T.R., & TERANISHI, R. (1984) Comparison of headspace volatiles from winged beans and soybeans. *J. agric. food Chem.*, 32: 1011-1015.

48. DE ZWART, D. & SLOOFF, W. (1983) The Microtox as an alternative assay in the acute toxicity assessment of water pollutants. *Aquat. Toxicol.*, 4: 129-138.

49. DORIGAN, J., FULLER, B., & DUFFY, R. (1976) *Scoring of organic air pollutants. Chemistry, production and toxicity of selected synthetic organic*

chemicals, The MITRE Corporation (MITRE Technical Report MTR-7248, Rev. 1, Appendix III).

50. DRAVNIEKS, A. (1974) A building-block model for the characterization of odorant molecules and their odors. *Ann. N.Y. Acad. Sci.*, **237**: 144-163.

51. DRY, I., WALLACE, W., & NICHOLAS, D.J.D. (1981) Role of ATP in nitrite reduction in roots of wheat and pea. *Planta*, **152**: 234-238.

52. DURWALD, W. & DEGEN, W. (1956) [A fatal poisoning by *n*-propyl alcohol.] *Arch. Toxikol.*, **16**: 84-88 (in German).

53. DUVEL, W.A. & HELFGOTT, T. (1975) Removal of wastewater organics by reverse osmosis. *J. Water Pollut. Control Fed.*, **47**: 57-65.

54. EICEMAN, G.A. & KARASEK, F.W. (1981) Identification of residual organic compounds in food packages. *J. Chromatogr.*, 210: 93-103.

55. FANG, H.H.P. & CHIAN, E.S.K. (1976) Reverse osmosis separation of polar organic compounds in aqueous solution. *Environ. Sci. Technol.*, 10: 364-369.

56. FAO/WHO (1980) *Toxicological evaluation of certain food additives.* Report of the Joint FAO/WHO Expert Committee on Food Additives, Geneva, World Health Organization, pp. 162-168 (WHO Food Additive Series 16).

57. FERNANDEZ, F. & QUIGLEY, R.M. (1985) Hydraulic conductivity of natural clays permeated with simple liquid hydrocarbons. *Can. geotech. J.*, **22**: 205-214.

58. FLATH, R.A., ALTIERI, M.A., & MON, T.R. (1984) Volatile constituents of *Amaranthus retroflexus* L. *J. agric. food Chem.*, **32**: 92-94.

59. FLICK, E.W. (1985) *Industrial solvents handbook.* New Jersey, Noyes Data Corp., pp. 220-223.

60. FORSANDER, O.A. (1967) Influence of some aliphatic alcohols on the metabolism of rat liver slices. *Biochem. J.*, **105**: 93-97.

61. GAD, S.C., DUNN ,B.J., DOBBS, D.W., REILLY, C., & WALSH, R.D. (1986) Development and validation of an alternative dermal sensitization test: the mouse ear swelling test (MEST). *Toxicol. appl. Pharmacol.*, **84**: 93-114.

62. GAGE, P.W. (1965) The effect of methyl, ethyl and *n*-propyl alcohol on neuromuscular transmission in the rat. *J. Pharmacol. exp. Ther.*, **150**: 236-243.

63. GAILLARD, D. & DERACHE, R. (1966) Action de quelques alcools aliphatiques sur la mobilisation de différentes fractions lipidiques chez le rat. *Food Cosmet. Toxicol.*, 4: 515-520.

64. GELSOMINI, N. (1985) Head-space analysis with capillary columns in quality control of wines. In: *Proceedings of the 6th International Symposium on Capillary Chromatography*, pp. 515-519.

65. GERARDE, H.W., AHLSTROM, D.B., & LINDEN, N.J. (1966) The aspiration hazard and toxicity of a homologous series of alcohols. *Arch. environ. Health*, 13: 457-461.

66. GERHOLD, R.M. & MALANEY, G.W. (1966) Structural determinants in the oxidation of aliphatic compounds by activated sludge. *J. Water Pollut. Control Fed.*, 38: 562-579.

67. GIBEL, W., LOHS, K., & WILDNER, G.P. (1975) [Experimental study on the cancerogenic activity of propanol-1, 2-methylpropanol-1 and 3-methylbutanol. I.] *Arch. Geschwulstforsch.*, 45: 19-24 (in German).

68. GILLETTE, L.A., MILLER, D.L., & REDMAN, H.E. (1952) Appraisal of a chemical waste problem by fish toxicity tests. *Sewage ind. Waste*, 24: 1397-1401.

69. GIUSTI, D.M., CONWAY, R.A., & LAWSON, C.T. (1974) Activated carbon adsorption of petrochemicals. *J. Water Pollut. Control Fed.*, 46: 947-965.

70. GLASGOW, A.M. & CHASE, H.P. (1976) Effect of propionic acid on fatty acid oxidation and ureagenesis. *Pediatr. Res.*, 10: 683-686.

71. GOODMAN, D.E. & RAO, R.M. (1984) GC determination of fusel alcohols in distilled alcoholic beverages. *Am. Lab.*, 16: 100-103.

72. GORESKY, C.A., GORDON, E.R., & BACH, G.G. (1983) Uptake of monohydric alcohols by liver: demonstration of a shared enzymic space. *Am. J. Physiol.*, 244: G198-G214.

73. GOTZ-SCHMIDT, E.-M. & SCHREIER, P. (1986) Neutral volatiles from blended endive (*Cichorium endivia* L.). *J. agric. food Chem.*, 34: 212-215.

74. GRANT, K.A. & SAMSON, H.H. (1984) *n*-Propanol induced microcephaly in the neonatal rat. *Neurobehav. Toxicol. Teratol.*, 6: 165-169.

75. GRAY, V.M. & CRESSWELL, C.F. (1983) The effect of respiratory inhibitors and alcohols on nitrate utilization and nitrite accumulation in excised roots of *Z. mays* L. *Z. Pflanzenphysiol.*, 112: 207-214.

76. GREGERSEN, N. (1979) Studies on the effects of saturated and unsaturated short-chain monocarboxylic acids on the energy metabolism of rat liver mitochondria. *Pediat. Res.*, 14: 1227-1230.

77. GREGERSEN, N. (1981) The specific inhibition of the pyruvate dehydrogenase complex from pig kidney by propionyl-CoA and isovaleryl-CoA. *Biochem. Med. III*, 26: 20-27.

78. GULATI, A., NATH, C., SHANKER, K., SRIMAL, R.C., DHAWAN, K.N., & BHARGAVA, K.P. (1985) Effects of alcohols on the permeability of blood-brain barrier. *Pharmacol. Res. Commun.*, 17: 85-93.

79. HANSSEN, H.-P., SPRECHER, E., & KLINGENBERG, A. (1984) Accumulation of volatile flavour compounds in liquid cultures of *Kluyveromyces lactis* strains. *Z. Naturforsch.*, 39c: 1030-1033.

80. HANSCH, C. & ANDERSON, S. (1967) The effect of intramolecular hydrophobic bonding on partition coefficients. *J. org. Chem.*, 32: 2583-2586.

81. HARRIS, R.A. (1983) Ethanol, membrane perturbation, and synaptosomal ion transport. *Proc. West. Pharmacol. Soc.*, 26: 255-257.

82. HAWLEY, G.G. (1981) *Condensed chemical dictionary*, 10th ed., Melbourne, Van Nostrand Reinhold Company Inc.

83. HELLMAN, T.M. & SMALL, F.H. (1974) Characterization of the odor properties of 101 petrochemicals using sensory methods. *J. Air Pollut. Control Assoc.*, 24: 979-982.

84. HERMENS, J., BUSSER, F., LEEUWANGH, P., & MUSCH, A. (1985) Quantitative structure-activity relationships and mixture toxicity of organic chemicals in *Photobacterium phosphoreum*: the Microtox 85 test. *Ecotoxicol. environ. Saf.*, 9: 17-25.

85. HILLBOM, M.E., FRANSSILA, K., & FORSANDER, O.A. (1974) Effects of chronic ingestion of some lower aliphatic alcohols in rats. *Res. Commun. chem. Pathol. Pharmacol.*, 9: 177-180.

86. HILSCHER, H., GEISSLER, E., LOHS, K., & GIBEL, W. (1969) [Studies on the toxicity and mutagenicity of single fusel oil components on *E. coli*.] *Acta biol. med. Germ.*, 23: 843-852 (in German).

87. HIRANO, K., WATANABE, Y., ADACHI, T., ITO, Y., & SUGIURA, M. (1985) Drug-binding properties of human α-foetoprotein. *Biochem J.*, 231: 189-191.

88. HO, Y.H., SCHWARZE, I., & SOEHRING, K. (1970) [The influence of low aliphatic alcohols on the chloral hydrate metabolism in rat liver sections.] *Arzneim.-Forsch.*, 20: 1507-1509 (in German).

89. HODGE, H.C. & STERNER, J.H. (1943) *Am. ind. Hyg. Assoc. Q.*, 10: 93.

90. HOIGNE, J. & BADER, H. (1983) Rate constants of reactions of ozone with organic and inorganic compounds in water. I. Non-dissociating organic compounds. *Water Res.*, 17: 173-183.

91. HORWITZ, W., ed. (1975) *Official methods of analysis of the Association of Official Analytical Chemists*, 12th ed., Washington DC, Association of Official Analytical Chemists, 161pp.

92. HOVIOUS, J.C., CONWAY, R.A., & GANZE, C.W. (1973) Anaerobic lagoon pretreatment of petrochemical wastes. *J. Water Pollut. Control Fed.*, 45: 71-84.

93. HUANG, R.-D, SMITH, M.F., & ZAHLER, W.L. (1982). Inhibition of Forskolin-activated adenylate cyclase by ethanol and other solvents. *J. cyclic Nucleotide Res.*, 8: 385-394.

94. HUDOLEI, V.V., MIZGIREV, I.V., & PLISS, G.B. (1987) [Evaluation of mutagenic activity of carcinogens and other chemical agents with *Salmonella typhimurium* assays.] *Vopr. Onkol.*, 32: 73-80 (in Russian).

95. IRPTC (1987) *Data profile on n-propanol*, Geneva, Switzerland, International Register of Potentially Toxic Chemicals, United Nations Environment Programme.

96. IVANETICH, K.M., LUCAS, S., MARSH, J.A., ZIMAN, M.R., KATZ, I.D., & BRADSHAW, J.J. (1978) Organic compounds. Their interaction with and degradation of hepatic microsomal drug-metabolizing enzymes *in vitro. Drug Metab. Dispos.*, 6: 218-225.

97. JADDOU, H.A., PAVEY, J.A., & MANNING, D.J. (1978) Chemical analysis of flavour volatiles in heat-treated milks. *J. dairy Res.*, 45: 391-403.

98. JOUANY, J.-P. (1982) Volatile fatty acid and alcohol determination in digestive contents, silage juices, bacterial cultures and anaerobic fermentor contents. *Sci. Aliment.*, 2: 131-144.

99. JUHNKE, I. & LUDEMANN, D. (1978) [Results of examination of 200 chemical compounds for acute toxicity towards fish by means of the golden orfe test.] *Z. Wasser-Abwasser Forsch.*, 11: 161-164 (in German).

100. KAMIL, I.A., SMITH, J.N., & WILLIAMS, R.T. (1953) The metabolism of aliphatic alcohols. The glucuronic acid conjugation of acyclic aliphatic alcohols. *Biochem. J.*, 53: 129-136.

101. KANE, L.E., DOMBROSKE, R., & ALARIE, Y. (1980) Evaluation of sensory irritation from some common industrial solvents. *Am. Ind. Hyg. Assoc. J.*, 41: 451- 455.

102. KHARE, M. & DONDERO, N.C. (1977) Fractionation and concentration from water of volatiles and organics on high vacuum system: examination of sanitary landfill leachate. *Environ. Sci. Technol.*, 11: 814-819.

103. KINLIN, T.E., MURALIDHARA, R., PITTET, A.O., SANDERSON, A., & WALRADT, J.P. (1972) Volatile components of roasted filberts. *J. agric. food Chem.*, **20**: 1021-1028.

104. KIRK, R.E & OTHMER, D.F., ed. (1978-1984) *Encyclopedia of chemical technology*, 3rd ed., New York, Wiley Interscience.

105. KLECKA, G.M., LANDI, L.P., & BODNER, K.M. (1985) Evaluation of the OECD activated sludge, respiration inhibition test. *Chemosphere*, **14**: 1239-1251.

106. KNUTH, M.L. & HOGLUND, M.D. (1984) Quantitative analysis of 68 polar compounds from ten chemical classes by direct aqueous injection gas chromatography. *J. Chromatogr.*, **285**: 153-160.

107. KRAMER, V.C., SCHNELL, D.J., & NICKERSON, K.W. (1983) Relative toxicity of organic solvents to *Aedes aegypti* larvae. *J. Invertebr. Pathol.*, **42**: 285-287.

108. KRISTIANSEN , U., HANSEN, L. NIELSEN, G.A., & HOLST, E. (1986) Sensory irritation and pulmonary irritation of cumene and *n*-propanol: Mechanisms of receptor activation and desensitization. *Acta pharmacol. toxicol.*, **59**: 60-72.

109. KRULL, I.S., SWARTZ, M., & DRISCOLL, J.N. (1984) Derivatizations for improved detection of alcohols by gas chromatography and photoionization detection. *Anal. Lett.*, **17**(A20): 2369-2384.

110. KUHNHOLZ, B. (1985) [Reflections concerning the analysis of free aliphatic alcohols in tissue.] *Blutalkohol*, **22**: 455-461 (in German).

111. LAING, D.G. (1975) A comparative study of the olfactory sensitivity of humans and rats. *Chem. Senses Flavor*, 1: 257-269.

112. LANGVARDT, P.W. & MELCHER, R. (1979) Simultaneous determination of polar and non-polar solvents in air using a two-phase desorption from charcoal. *Am. Ind. Hyg. Assoc. J.*, **40**: 1006-1012.

113. LASNE, C., GU, Z.W., VENEGAS, W., & CHOUROULINKOV, I. (1984) The *in vitro* micronucleus assay for detection of cytogenetic effects induced by mutagen-carcinogens: comparison with the *in vitro* sister-chromatid exchange assay. *Mutat. Res.*, **130**: 273-282.

114. LIEBICH, H.M., BUELOW, H.J., & KALLMAYER, R. (1982) Quantification of endogenous aliphatic alcohols in serum and urine. *J. Chromatogr.*, **239**: 343-349.

115. LUDWIG, E. & HAUSEN, B.M. (1977) Sensitivity to isopropyl alcohol. *Contact Dermatit.*, 3: 240-244.

116. LUTHIN, G.R. & TABAKOFF, B. (1984) Activation of adenylate cyclase by alcohols requires the nucleotide-binding protein. *J. Pharmacol. exp. Ther.*, **228**: 579-587.

117. LYON, R.C., MCCOMB, J.A., SCHREURS, J., & GOLDSTEIN, D.B. (1981) A relationship between alcohol intoxication and the disordering of brain membranes by a series of short-chain alcohols. *J. Pharmacol. exp. Ther.*, **218**: 669-675.

118. MAICKEL, R.P. & NASH, J.F. (1985) Differing effects of short-chain alcohols on body temperature and coordinated muscular activity in mice. *Neuropharmacology*, **24**: 83-89.

119. MCCREERY, M.J. & HUNT, W.A. (1978) Physico-chemical correlates of alcohol intoxication. *Neuropharmacology*, **17**: 451-461.

120. MANKES, R.F., LEFEVRE, R., RENAK,V., FIESHER, J., & ABRAHAM, R. (1985) Reproductive effects of some solvent alcohols with differing partition coefficients. *Teratology*, **31**: 67A.

121. MATSUI, F., LOVERING, E.G., WATSON, J.R., BLACK, D.B., & SEARS, R.W. (1984) Gas chromatographic method for solvent residues in drug raw materials. *J. pharm. Sci.*, **73**: 1664-1666.

122. MAY, J. (1966) [Odour thresholds of solvents for the judgement of solvent odour in air.] *Staub Reinhalt. Luft*, **26**: 385-389 (in German).

123. MAY, W.A., PETERSON, R.J., & CHANG, S.S. (1983) Chemical reactions involved in the deep-fat frying of foods. IX. Identification of the volatile decomposition products. *J. Am. Oil Chem. Soc.*, **60**: 990-995.

124. MICHAELIS, M.L. & MICHAELIS, E.K. (1983) Alcohol and local anesthetic effects on Na^+-dependent Ca^{2+}-fluxes in brain synaptic membrane vesicles. *Biochem. Pharmacol.*, **32**: 963-969.

125. MIKHEEV, M.J., & FROLOVA, A.D. (1978) [Toxicokinetics of certain representatives of a homologous series of alcohols.] *Gig. i Sanit.*, **6**:33-36 (in Russian).

126. MORGAN, E.T., KOOP, D.R., & COON, M.J. (1982) Catalytic activity of cytochrome P-450 isozyme 3a isolated from liver microsomes of ethanol-treated rabbits. *J. biol. Chem.*, **257**: 13951-13957.

127. MOSHONAS, M.G. & SHAW, P.E. (1987) Quantitative analysis of orange juice flavor volatiles by direct-injection gas chromatography. *J. Agric. food Chem.*, **35**:161-165.

129. MULLIN, M.J. & HUNT, W.A. (1985) Actions of ethanol on voltage-sensitive sodium channels: effects on neurotoxin-stimulated sodium uptake in synaptosomes. *J. Pharmacol. exp. Ther.*, **232**: 413-419.

130. MUNCH, J.C. (1972) Aliphatic alcohols and alkyl esters: narcotic and lethal potencies to tadpoles and to rabbits. *Ind. Med.*, 41: 31-33.

131. MURPHREE, H.B., GREENBERG, L.A., & CARROLL, R.B. (1967) Neuropharmacological effects of substances other than ethanol in alcoholic beverages. *Fed. Proc.*, **26**: 1468-1473.

132. NELSON, B.K., BRIGHTWELL, W.S., & BURG, J.R. (1985) Comparison of behavioural teratogenic effects of ethanol and *n*-propanol administered by inhalation to rats. *Neurobehav. Toxicol Teratol.*, **7**: 770-783.

132. NELSON, B.K., BRIGHTWELL, W.S., MACKENZIE- TAYLOR, D.R., KHAN, A., BURG, J.R., WEIGEL, W.W. & GOAD, P.T. (1988) Teratogenicity of *n*-propanol and isopropanol administered at high inhalation concentration to rats. *Food Chem. Toxicol.*, **26**(3):247-254.

133. NEY, K.H. (1985) [Flavour of Tilsit cheese.] *Fette Seifen Anstrichmittel*, **87**: 289-293 (in German).

134. NGUYEN, V.C. & KATO, H. (1982) Volatile flavor components of Kumazasa (*Sasa albo-marginata*). *Agric. Biol. Chem.*, **46** : 2795-2801.

135. NUNOMURA, N., SASAKI, M., & YOKOTSUKA, T. (1984) Shoyu (soy sauce) flavor components: neutral fraction. *Agric. Biol. Chem.*, **48**: 1753-1762.

136. OBE, G. & RISTOW, H. (1977) Acetaldehyde, but not ethanol, induces sister chromatid exchanges in Chinese hamster cells *in vitro. Mutat. Res.*, **56**: 211- 213.

137. ODKVIST, L.M., LARSBY, B., THAM, R., & ASCHAN, G. (1979) On the mechanism of vestibular disturbances caused by industrial solvents. *Adv. Oto-Rhino-Laryng.*, **25**: 167-172.

138. OELERT, H.H. & FLORIAN, T. (1972) [Recording and valuation of the inconvenience caused by odours from diesel exhaust.] *Staub. Reinhalt. Luft*, **32**: 400-407 (in German).

139. OERSKOV, S.I. (1950) Experiments on the oxydation of propyl alcohol in rabbits. *Acta physiol. Scand.*, **20**: 258-262.

140. OTSUK141.A, K., IKI, I., & YAMASHITA, T. (1979) [Relationship between type of whisky and volatile component.] *Hakkokogaku*, **57**: 20-30 (in Japanese).

141. OVEREND, R. & PARASKEVOPOULOS, G. (1978) Rates of OH radical reactions. 4. Reactions with methanol, ethanol, 1-propanol, and 2-propanol at 296 K. *J. phys. Chem.*, **82**: 1329-1333.

142. PALO, V. & ILKOVA, H. (1970) Direct gas chromatographic estimation of lower alcohols, acetaldehyde, acetone and diacetyl in milk products. *J. Chromatogr.*, **53**: 363-367.

143. PATERNOSTRE, M., PICHON, Y., & DUPEYRAT, M. (1983) Effects of n-alcohols on ionic transmembrane currents in the squid giant axon. *Stud. phys. thero. Chem.*, **24**: 515-522.

144. PITTER, P. (1976) Determination of biological degradability of organic substances. *Water Res.*, **10**: 231-235.

145. POSO, H. & POSO, A.R. (1980) Inhibition by aliphatic alcohols of the stimulated activity of ornithine decarboxylase and tyrosine aminotransferase occurring in regenerating rat liver. *Biochem. Pharmacol.*, **29**: 2799-2803.

146. POSTEL, W. & ADAM, L. (1978) [Gas chromatographic characterization of whisky. III. Communication: Irish whiskey.] *Branntweinwirtsch.*, **118**: 404-407 (in German).

147. POWIS, G. (1975) Effect of a single oral dose of methanol, ethanol and propan-2-ol on the hepatic microsomal metabolism of foreign compounds in the rat. *Biochem. J.*, **148**: 269-277.

148. PREUSS, A. & ZIPFEL, K. (1985) [Headspace-gas chromatographic identification of alcoholic beverages and foodstuffs.] *Lebensmittelchem. gerichtl. Chem.*, **39**: 97-99 (in German).

149. PRICE, K.S., WAGGY, G.T., & CONWAY, R.A. (1974) Brine shrimp bioassay and seawater BOD of petrochemicals. *J. Water Pollut. Control Fed.*, **46**: 63-77.

150. PRIESTLEY, D.A. & LEOPOLD, A.C. (1980) Alcohol stress on soya bean seeds. *Ann. Bot.*, **45**: 39-45.

151. PUNTER, P.H. (1983) Measurement of human olfactory thresholds for several groups of structurally related compounds. *Chem. Senses*, 7: 215-235.

152. PURCHASE, I.F.H. (1969) Studies in kaffircorn malting and brewing. XXII. The acute toxicity of some fusel oils found in Bantu beer. *S.A. med. J.*, **43**: 795-798.

153. QUISTAD, G.B., STAIGER, L.E. & SCHOOLEY, D.A. (1986) The role of carnitine in the conjugation of acidic xenobiotics. *Drug Metab. Dispos.*, 14:521-525.

154. RAMSEY, J.D. & FLANAGAN, R.J. (1982) Detection and identification of volatile organic compounds in blood by headspace gas chromatograpy as an aid to the diagnosis of solvent abuse. *J. Chromatogr.*, **240**: 423-444.

155. REQUENA, J., VELAZ, M.E., GUERRERO, J.R., & MEDINA, J.D. (1985) Isomers of long-chain alkane derivatives and nervous impulse blockage. *J. membr. Biol.*, **84**: 229-238.

156. REYNOLDS, T. (1977) Comparative effects of aliphatic compounds on inhibition of lettuce fruit germination. *Ann. Bot.*, **41**: 637-648.

157. RIETBROCK, N. & ABSHAGEN, U. (1971) [Pharmacokinetics and metabolism of aliphatic alcohols.] *Arzneim.-Forsch.*, **21**: 1309-1319 (in German).

158. ROE, C.R., MILLINGTON, D.S., MALTBY, D.A., BOHAN, T.P. & HOPPEL, C.L. (1984) L-Carnitine enhances excretion of propionyl coenzyme A as propionylcarnitine in propionic acidemia. *J. clin. Invest.* **73**:1785-1788.

159. ROSS, D.H. (1976) Selective action of alcohols on cerebral calcium levels. *Ann. N.Y. Acad. Sci.*, **273**: 280-294.

160. RYAN, D.E., THOMAS, P.E., WRIGHTON, S.A., GUZELIAN, P.S. & LEVIN, W. (1987) Ethanol-inducible rat and human liver cytochrome P-450: characterization and role as high affinity N-nitrosodimethylamine demethylamine demethylases. In: Miners, J., Birkett, D.J., Drew, R., May, B., & McManus, ed. *Microsomes and drug oxidations*, London, Taylor & Francis, pp. 3-11.

161. SABLJIC, A. & PROTIC-SABLIC, M. (1983) Quantitative structure-activity study on the mechanism of inhibition of microsomal *p*-hydroxylation of aniline by alcohols. *Mol. Pharmacol.*, **23**: 213-218.

162. SAHU, B.R. & TANDON, U. (1983) A novel method for spot test detection of alcohols. *J. Indian Chem. Soc.*, **60**: 615-616.

163. SANCEDA, N., KURATA, T., & ARAKAWA, N. (1984) Fractionation and identification of volatile compounds in Patis, a Phillipine fish sauce. *Agric. Biol. Chem.*, **48**: 3047-3052.

164. SAVINI, E.C. (1968) Estimation of the LD_{50} in mol/kg. *Proc. Eur. Soc. Study Drug Toxicol.*, **9**: 276-278.

165. SCHEIMAN, M.A., SAUNDERS, R.A., & SAALFELD, F.E. (1974) Organic contaminants in the District of Columbia water supply. *Biomed. Mass Spectrom.*, **1**: 209-211.

166. SCOTT, T. & EAGLESON, M. (1983) *Concise encyclopedia of biochemistry.* New York, W. de Gruyter, pp. 158-159.

167. SEILER, H., BLAIM, H., & BUSSE, M. (1984) [Antibacterial effects on predominant taxa in the activated sludge system of a chemical combine.] *Z. Wasser-Abwasser Forsch.*, **17**: 127-133 (in German).

168. SHAW, G.J., ALLEN, J.M., & VISSER, F.R. (1985) Volatile flavor components of Babaco fruit (*Carica pentagona* Heilborn). *J. agric. food Chem.*, 33: 795-797.

169. SINCLAIR, J.F., SMITH, L., BEMENT, W.J., SINCLAIR, P.R., & BONKOWSKY, H.L. (1982) Increases in cytochrome P-450 in cultured hepatocytes mediated by 3- and 4-carbon alcohols. *Biochem. Pharmacol.*, 31: 2811-2815.

170. SLOOFF, W. (1983) Benthic macroinvertebrates and water quality assessment: some toxicological considerations. *Aquat. Toxicol.*, 4 : 73-82.

171. SLOOFF, W. & BAERSELMAN, R. (1980) Comparison of the usefulness of the Mexican Axolotl (*Ambystoma mexicanum*) and the clawed toad (*Xenopus laevis*) in toxicological bioassays. *Bull. environ. Contam. Toxicol.*, 24: 439-443.

172. SLOOFF, W., CANTON, J.H., & HERMENS, J.L.M. (1983) Comparison of the susceptibility of 22 freshwater species to 15 chemical compounds. I. (Sub)acute toxicity tests. *Aquat. Toxicol.*, 4: 113-128.

173. SMYTH, H.F., CARPENTER, C.P., WEIL, C.S., & POZZANI, U.C. (1954) Range-finding toxicity data. *Arch. ind. Hyg. occup. Med.*, 10: 61-68.

174. SNIDER, J.B. & DAWSON, G.A. (1985) Tropospheric light alcohols, carbonyls, and acetonitrile: concentrations in the southwestern United States and Henry's law data. *J. geophys. Res.*, 90: 3797-3805.

175. SOLIMAN, M.A., EL SAWY, A.A., FADEL, H.M., OSMAN, F., & GAD, A.M. (1985) Volatile components of roasted *Citrillus colocynthis*, var. Colocynthoides. *Agric. Biol. Chem.*, 49: 269- 275.

176. SRI (1984) *n*-Propanol: record number 0115 (last revision date 01-06-84). In: *Toxicology data bank*, Palo Alto, California, Stanford Research Institute, Bethesda, Maryland, National Library of Medicine.

177. STENSTROM, S., ENLOE, L., PFENNING, M., & RICHELSON, E. (1986) Acute effects of ethanol and other short-chain alcohols on the guanylate cyclase system of murine neuroblastoma cells (clone N1E-115). *J. Pharmacol. exp. Ther.*, 236: 458-463.

178. STOCK, K. & SCHMIDT, M. (1978) Effects of short-chain alcohols on adenylate cyclase in plasma membranes of rat adipocytes. *Naunyn-Schmiedeberg Arch. Pharmacol.*, 302: 37-43.

179. STOFBERG, J. & GRUNDSCHOBER, F. (1984) Consumption ratio and food predominance of flavoring materials: second cumulative series. *Perfumer Flavorist*, 9: 53-83.

180. STOKES, J.A. & HARRIS, R.A. (1982) Alcohols and synaptosomal calcium transport. *Mol. Pharmacol.*, 22: 99-104.

181. STOLZENBERG, S.J. & HINE, C.H. (1979) Mutagenicity of halogenated and oxygenated three-carbon compounds. *J. Toxicol. environ. Health*, **5**: 1149-1158.

182. STONE, H., PRYOR, G.T., & STEINMETZ, G. (1972) A comparison of olfactory adaptation among seven odorants and their relationship with several physico-chemical properties. *Perception Psychophys.*, **12**: 501-504.

183. STRANGE, A.W., SCHNEIDER, C.W., & GOLDBORT, R. (1976) Selection of C_3 alcohols by high and low ethanol selecting mouse strains and the effects on open field activity. *Pharmacol. Biochem. Behav.*, **4**: 527-530.

184. STUMPF, D.A., MCAFEE, J., PARKS, J.K., & EGUREN, L. (1986) Propionate inhibition of succinate: CoA ligase (GDP) and the citric acid cycle in mitochondria. *Pediatr. Res.*, **14**: 1127-1131.

185. TABAKOFF, B. & HOFFMAN, P.L. (1983) Alcohol interactions with brain opiate receptors. *Life Sci.*, **32**: 197-204.

186. TANDOI, P., GUIDOTTI, M., & STACCHINI, P. (1984) [On the composition of brandies.] *Riv. Soc. Ital. Sci. Aliment.*, **13**: 69-76 (in Italian).

187. TAYLOR, J.M., JENNER, P.M., & JONES, W.I. (1964) A comparison of the toxicity of some allyl, propenyl, and propyl compounds in the rat. *Toxicol. appl. Pharmacol.*, **6**: 378-387.

188. TESCHKE, R., HASUMURA, Y., & LIEBER, C.S. (1975) Hepatic microsomal alcohol-oxidizing system. Affinity for methanol, ethanol, propanol, and butanol. *J. biol. Chem.*, **250**: 7397-7403.

189. TESTA, B. (1981) Structural and electronic factors influencing the inhibition of aniline hydroxylation by alcohols and their binding to cytochrome P-450. *Chem.-biol. Interact.*, **34**: 287- 300.

190. TICHY, M., TRCKA, V. ROTH, Z., & KRIVUCOVA, M. (1985) QSAR analysis and data extrapolation among mammals in a series of aliphatic alcohols. *Environ. Health Perspect.*, **61**: 321-328.

191. TOMERA, J.F., SKIPPER, P.L., WISHNOK, J.S., TANNEBAUM, S.R., & BRUNENGRABER, H. (1984) Inhibition of N-nitroso-dimethylamine metabolism by ethanol and other inhibitors in the isolated perfused rat liver. *Carcinogenesis*, **5**: 113-116.

192. UHLEMANN, E.R., ROBBERECHT, P., & GARDNER, J.D. (1979) Effects of alcohols on the actions of VIP and secretin on acinar cells from guinea-pig pancreas. *Gastroenterology*, **76**: 917-925.

193. UNRUH, J.D. & SPINICELLI, L. (1981) Propyl alcohols, n-propyl alcohol. In: Kirk, R.E. & Othmer, D.F., ed. *Encyclopedia of chemical technology*, 3rd ed., New York, Wiley Interscience, Vol. 19, pp. 221-227,194.

194. URANO, K., OGURA, K., & WADA, H. (1981) Direct analytical method for aliphatic compounds in water by steam carrier gas chromatography. *Water Res.*, 15: 225-231.

195. US NIOSH (1984) Method 1401. In: Eller, P.M., ed. *NIOSH Manual of analytical methods*, 3rd ed., Cincinnati, Ohio, National Institute for Occupational Safety and Health, Vol. 1, pp. 1401-1-1401-4.

196. VAISHNAV, D.D. & LOPAS, D.M. (1985) Relationship between lipophilicity and biodegradation inhibition of selected industrial chemicals. *Dev. ind. Microbiol.*, 26: 557-565.

197. VEITH, G.D. & KOSIAN, P. (1983) Estimating bioconcentration potential from octanol/water partition coefficients. In: Mackay et al., ed. *Physical behaviour of PCBs in the Great Lakes*, Ann Arbor, Michigan, Ann Arbor Science, pp. 269-282.

198. VERSCHUEREN, K. (1983) *Handbook of environmental data on organic chemicals*, 2nd ed., Melbourne, Van Nostrand Reinhold Company Inc.

199. VIDELA, L.A., FERNANDEZ, V., & DE MARINIS, A. (1982) Liver peroxidative pressure and glutathione status following acetaldehyde and aliphatic alcohols pretreatment in the rat. *Biochem. Biophys. Res. Commun.*, 104: 965-970.

200. VON DER HUDE, W., SCHEUTWINKEL, M., GRAMLICH, U., FISSLER, B., & BASLER, A. (1987) Genotoxicity of three carbon compounds evaluated in the SCE test *in vitro*. *Environ. Mutagen.*, 9: 401-410.

201. WACHTEL, R.E. (1984) Aliphatic alcohols increase the decay rate of glutamate-activated currents at the crayfish neuromuscular junction. *Br. J. Pharmacol.*, 83: 393-397.

202. WAGNER, R. (1976) [Investigations into the degradation behaviour of organic compounds using the respirometric dilution method. II. The degradation kinetics of the test compounds.] *Vom Wasser*, 47: 241-265.

203. WAKABAYASHI, T., HORIUCHI, M., SAKAGUCHI, M., ONDA, H., & IIJIMA, M. (1984) Induction of megamitochondria in the rat liver by n-propyl alcohol and n-butyl alcohol. *Acta pathol. Jpn.*, 34: 471-480.

204. WALLGREN, H. (1960) Relative intoxicating effects on rats of ethyl, propyl and butyl alcohols. *Acta pharmacol. toxicol.*, 16: 217-222.

205. WATERER, D.R. & PRITCHARD, M.K. (1985a) Volatile production by wounded Russet Burbank and Norland potatoes. *Sci. Aliments*, 5: 205-216.

206. WATERER, D.R. & PRITCHARD, M.K. (1985b) Production of volatile metabolites in potatoes infected by *Erwinia carotovora* var. carotovora and *E. carotovora* var. atroseptica. *Can. J. plant Pathol.*, 7: 47-51.

207. WILKIN, J.K. & FORTNER, G. (1985) Cutaeous vascular sensitivity to lower aliphatic alcohols and aldehydes in orientals. *Alcoholism clin. exp. Res.,* **9**: 522-525.

208. WINTERSTEIGER, R., GAMSE, G., & PACHA, W. (1982) [Quantification of alcoholic compounds and amines with 4-(6-methylbenzo-thiazol-2-yl)phenyl isocyanate. *Fresenius Z. anal. Chem.,* **312**: 455-461.

209. WOLF, M., URBÀN, R., WELLER, J.-P., & TROGER, H.D. (1985) [The analysis of congeners of alcoholic beverages in blood. First communication: the application of capillary gas chromatography in micro head-space analysis.] *Blutalkohol,* **22**: 321-332 (in German).

210. WOLFF, T. (1978) *In vitro* inhibition of monooxygenase dependent reactions by organic solvents. *Int. Congr. Ser. Excerpta Med.,* **440**: 196-199.

211. YAJIMA, I., YANAI, T., NAKAMURA, M., SAKAKIBARA, H., UCHIDA, H., & HAYASHI, K. (1983) Volatile flavor compounds of boiled buckwheat flour. *Agric. Biol. Chem.,* **47**: 729-738.

212. YAJIMA, I., YANAI, T., NAKAMURA, M., SAKAKIBARA, H., & HAYASHI, K. (1984) Volatile flavor components of Kogyoku apples. *Agric. Biol. Chem.,* **48**: 849-855.

213. YASHUDA, Y., CABRAL, A.M., & ANTONIO, A. (1976) Inhibitory action of aliphatic alcohols on smooth muscle contraction. *Pharmacology,* **14**: 473-478.

214. YASUHARA, A. & FUWA, K. (1982) Characterization of odorous compounds in rotten blue-green algae. *Agric. Biol. Chem.,* **46**: 1761-1766.

215. YASUHARA, A., FUWA, K., & JIMBU, M. (1984) Identification of odorous compounds in fresh and rotten swine manure. *Agric. Biol. Chem.,* **48**: 3001-3010.

216. YOUNG, P.J. & PARKER, A. (1983) The identification and possible environmental impact of trace gases and vapours in landfill gas. *Waste Manag. Res.,* **1**: 213-226.

RESUME

1. Identité, propriétés physiques et chimiques, méthodes d'analyse

Le propanol-1 est un liquide incolore, très inflammable, qui est volatil à la température ambiante et sous la pression atmosphérique normale. Il est miscible à l'eau et aux solvants organiques. Parmi les méthodes d'analyse, on peut citer la chromatographie en phase gazeuse, qui permet de déceler jusqu'à 5×10^{-5} mg/m^3 dans l'air, 1×10^{-4} mg/litre dans l'eau et 0,002 mg/litre dans le sang, le sérum ou les urines lorsque l'échantillon a été extrait ou concentré de façon satisfaisante.

2. Sources d'exposition humaine et environnementale

La capacité de production mondiale a dépassé 130 000 tonnes en 1979. Le propanol-1 d'origine naturelle résulte de la décomposition de matériaux organiques par divers microorganismes et on le rencontre également dans les végétaux et le mazout. Industriellement, on le produit par réaction de l'éthylène sur l'oxyde de carbone et l'hydrogène qui donne du propionaldéhyde, celui-ci étant ensuite hydrogéné en propanol. C'est également un sous-produit de la fabrication du méthanol et il peut être obtenu directement à partir du propane ou de l'acroléine. Le propanol-1 est essentiellement un solvant à tout faire, à usage industriel ou domestique. Il entre dans la composition des encres d'imprimerie flexographiques et il est également utilisé dans l'industrie textile, dans des produits à usage personnel tels que les produits cosmétiques, les lotions ainsi que dans les produits pour le nettoyage des vitres, les encaustiques et les antiseptiques. En second lieu par ordre d'importance, on peut citer son utilisation comme produit intermédiaire dans la fabrication de divers composés chimiques.

3. Transport, distribution et transformation dans l'environnement

La principale voie de pénétration de propanol-1 dans l'environnement est constituée par les émissions dans l'atmosphère qui se produisent au cours de la production, de la transformation, du stockage, du transport et de l'utilisation de ce composé ou du rejet de déchets qui en contiennent. Il peut y avoir également des décharges dans l'eau et le sol. Le propanol-1 étant principalement utilisé comme solvant volatil, il finit par se dissiper en grande partie dans l'environnement.

Le propanol-1 est rapidement éliminé de l'atmosphère par réaction sur les radicaux hydroxyles et par les précipitations. Il est facilement biodégradable tant par voie aérobie que par voie anaérobie et du fait de l'existence de ces mécanismes d'élimination chimique et biologique, on ne le rencontre normalement pas en quantité mesurable dans l'environnement. Toutefois on en a décelé la présence dans l'air des agglomérations urbaines, dans des décharges, ainsi que dans les eaux s'échappant de zones d'enfouissement de déchets.

Le logarithme du coefficient de partage n-octanol/eau du propanol-1 est de 0,34 et son facteur de bioconcentration a une valeur de 0,7, ce qui en rend la bioaccumulation très improbable.

4. Niveau dans l'environnement et exposition humaine

La population en général peut être exposée au propanol par suite d'une ingestion accidentelle, par inhalation lors de l'utilisation du produit ou par absorption avec la nourriture (propanol d'origine naturelle, additif d'aromatisation ou reste de solvant) ou des boissons alcoolisées ou non. Par exemple la bière en contient jusqu'à 195 mg/litre, le vin jusqu'à 116 mg/litre et certains spiritueux jusqu'à 3500 mg/litre. L'exposition de la population par suite d'inhalation ou de la consommation d'eau de boisson est faible (aux Etats-Unis la concentration moyenne dans des échantillons d'air urbain se situait à 0,00005 mg/m^3 et dans des échantillons d'eau de boisson, à 0,001 mg/litre). Les travailleurs courent un risque d'exposition par inhalation lors de la production, de la transformation et de l'utilisation du produit. Toutefois, on ne dispose d'aucune donnée qui permettrait de chiffrer ce type d'exposition.

5. Cinétique et métabolisme

Après ingestion, le propanol-1 est rapidement absorbé et distribué dans l'ensemble de l'organisme. On manque de données sur la vitesse d'absorption après inhalation et exposition cutanée. Le propanol-1 est métabolisé par l'alcool déshydrogénase (ADH) en aldéhyde puis acide propionique et peut entrer dans le cycle de Krebs. Cette oxydation constitue l'étape limitante du métabolisme du propanol-1. *In vitro,* les oxydases microsomiques du rat et du lapin sont également capables d'oxyder le propanol-1 en aldéhyde propionique. L'ADH et des systèmes d'oxydation microsomiques ont une affinité beaucoup plus importante pour le propanol-1 que pour l'éthanol; aussi le propanol-1 est-il rapidement éliminé de l'organisme. Chez le rat, sa demi-vie après administration par voie orale d'une dose de 1000 mg/kg est de 45 minutes.

Chez l'animal et chez l'homme, le propanol-1 peut être éliminé de l'organisme dans l'air expiré ou dans les urines. Chez des êtres humains ayant reçu par voie orale une dose de 3,75 mg de propanol-1 par kg de poids corporel et de 1200 mg d'éthanol par kg de poids corporel, l'excrétion urinaire totale du propanol-1 a été de 2,1 % de la dose. Les concentrations urinaires de propanol-1 étaient d'autant plus basses que la quantité d'éthanol ingérée simultanément était basse, ce qui montre qu'il y avait compétition pour l'ADH entre le propanol-1 et la surdose d'éthanol.

6. Effets sur les êtres vivant dans leur milieu naturel

Aux concentrations normalement présentes dans l'environnement, le propanol-1 n'est pas toxique pour la vie aquatique, les insectes ou les végétaux. Chez trois des espèces aquatiques les plus sensibles (trois protozoaires), le seuil l'inhibition de la multiplication cellulaire se situait entre 38 et 568 mg/litre. Dans le cas d'organismes plus évolués, la concentration létale était d'environ 5000 mg/litre, avec des variations remarquablement faibles d'un phylum à l'autre et une courbe dose-réponse de très forte pente. Certaines bactéries et micro-organismes qui vivent dans les eaux résiduaires et les boues activées sont capables de s'adapter à des concentrations supérieures à 17 000 mg/litre.

Le propanol-1 peut inhiber ou au contraire stimuler la germination des semences selon sa concentration dans l'eau d'arrosage et les conditions d'exposition. Le composé accroît l'accumulation de nitrites dans le maïs, les pois et le froment.

7. Effets sur les animaux d'expérience et sur les systèmes d'épreuve *in vitro*

Le propanol-1 présente une faible toxicité aiguë pour les mammifères (mesurée d'après la mortalité), que l'exposition se fasse par voie percutanée, orale ou respiratoire. On a fait état de valeurs allant de 1870 à 6800 mg par kg de poids corporel pour la DL$_{50}$ par voie orale chez plusieurs espèces animales. Toutefois pour de très jeunes rats, on donne une DL$_{50}$ orale de 560 à 660 mg par kg de poids corporel. Après une seule exposition, le principal effet toxique du propanol-1 consiste dans la dépression du système nerveux central. Selon les données disponibles, le propanol-1 exercerait sur le système nerveux central des effets analogues à ceux de l'éthanol; toutefois il semblerait que la neurotoxicité du propanol-1 soit plus importante. Les DE$_{50}$ pour l'anesthésie chez le lapin et la perte du réflexe de redressement chez la souris se situaient respectivement à 1440 mg par kg de poids corporel par voie orale et à 1478 mg par kg de poids corporel par voie intra-péritonéale; ces doses sont environ quatre fois plus faibles que dans le cas de l'éthanol. Dans l'épreuve du plan incliné, le propanol-1 s'est révélé 2,5 fois plus actif que l'éthanol chez le rat.

Des doses uniques de 3000 ou 6000 mg par kg de poids corporel administrées par voie orale à des rats ont provoqué une accumulation réversible de triglycérides dans le foie. Les vapeurs fortement concentrées provoquent une irritation des voies respiratoires chez la souris. Aux concentrations d'environ 30 000 mg/m^3 on note une réduction de 50 % du rythme respiratoire chez la souris.

On ne dispose de données ni sur l'irritation oculaire ni sur l'irritation cutanée. Aucun effet n'a été observé lors d'une épreuve de sensibilisation cutanée sur des souris CF1.

Chez des rats mâles exposés pendant six semaines à une dose de 15 220 mg/m^3 de propanol-1, on a relevé quelques signes d'une action nocive possible sur la fonction de reproduction. En revanche aucun effet n'a été noté à la dose de 8610 mg/m^3. Après exposition de rattes gravides au propanol-1, on a observé des signes patents de toxicité pour les mères et les foetus aux doses de 23 968 et 14 893 mg/m^3 (9743 et 6054 ppm respectivement); aucun signe de toxicité n'a été noté à 9001 mg/m^3 (3659 ppm). On n'a observé aucune anomalie comportementale parmi les descendants de rats mâles exposés pendant six semaines à 8610 ou 15 220 mg de propanol-1 par m^3, ni dans la descendance de rattes exposées pendant leur gestation aux mêmes concentrations. Toutefois, en administrant à des ratons de 5 à 8 jours des doses orales de 3000 à 7800 mg de propanol-1 par kg et par jour, on constatait des signes de dépression du SNC pendant l'administration et un syndrome de sevrage à la cessation du traitement. Le cerveau de ces rats a été examiné à l'âge de 18 jours; on a constaté une réduction du poids de cet organe tant en valeur absolue qu'en valeur relative, avec diminution de la teneur en ADN et réduction localisée des taux de cholestérol et de protéine.

La recherche de mutations ponctuelles au moyen de 2 épreuves utilisant *Salmonella typhimurium* n'a donné que des résultats négatifs, de même la recherche de mutations réverses sur *Escherichia coli* CA-274. Les résultats ont été également négatifs en ce qui concerne les échanges entre chromatides soeurs ou la présence de micro-noyaux dans les cellules mammaliennes *in vitro*. Il n'existe pas d'autres données relatives à la mutagénicité.

Lors d'une étude de cancérogénicité portant sur de petits groupes de rats Wistar exposés tout au long de leur existence par voie orale à des doses de 240 mg/kg ou par voie sous cutanée à des doses de 48 mg/kg, on a constaté un accroissement sensible de l'incidence des sarcomes du foie dans le groupe recevant le produit par voie sous cutanée. Toutefois cette étude ne permet pas d'apprécier la cancérogénicité du propanol-1, notamment à cause de l'absence de détails expérimentaux, du nombre trop restreint d'animaux et de l'utilisation d'une dose hépatotoxique unique très élevée.

8. Effets sur la santé humaine

On n'a pas signalé d'effets nocifs sur la santé humaine dans la population en général ou parmi des groupes professionnels. Le seul cas d'intoxication mortelle qui ait été signalé est celui d'une femme, retrouvée inconsciente et qui est décédé 4 à 5 heures après l'ingestion de propanol. L'autopsie a révélé un oedème cérébral et pulmonaire. Lors d'une étude sur l'irritation et la sensibilisation cutanées, on a signalé des réactions allergiques chez un membre du personnel du laboratoire. Chez neuf volontaires sur 12, on a observé un érythème qui a duré au moins 1 h après 5 minutes d'application sur les avant-bras de papiers filtres imprégnés de 0,025 ml d'une solution aqueuse à 75 % de propanol-1. On ne dispose d'aucun autre rapport concernant d'éventuels effets toxiques après exposition professionnelle au propanol-1.

Il n'existe pas d'études épidémiologiques qui permettent d'établir les effets à long terme, et notamment la cancérogénicité, du propanol-1 chez l'homme.

9. Résumé de l'évaluation

Il peut y avoir exposition humaine au propanol-1 à la suite de l'absorption de nourriture ou de boissons qui en contiennent. Une exposition par inhalation peut se produire lors de l'utilisation de ce produit à des fins ménagères, ou professionnelles, au cours de la fabrication, de la transformation et de l'utilisation de ce produit. Les données très limitées dont on dispose sur la teneur de l'air ambiant et de l'eau en propanol-1 indiquent que ces teneurs sont très faibles.

Le propanol-1 est rapidement absorbé et se répartit dans tout l'organisme après ingestion. Après inhalation, l'absorption est également rapide mais la résorption percutanée devrait être lente.

Chez l'animal, la toxicité aiguë du propanol-1 est faible, que l'exposition ait lieu par voie percutanée, par voir orale ou par voie respiratoire. L'exposition de personnes appartenant à la population générale à des teneurs potentiellement mortelles peut se produire à la suite d'une ingestion accidentelle ou volontaire. Toutefois, un seul cas d'intoxication mortelle par le propanol-1 a été signalé jusqu'ici. Les effets aigus les plus probables chez l'homme sont une intoxication de type alcoolique pouvant entraîner une narcose. L'expérimentation animale montre que le propanol-1 est 2 à 4 fois plus toxique que l'éthanol.

Le propanol-1 peut être irritant pour la peau mouillée.

On ne dispose pas de données suffisantes sur la toxicité chez l'animal pour procéder à une évaluation des risques pour la santé humaine qui découleraient d'une exposition répétée ou prolongée au propanol-1. Toutefois, un certain nombre d'études à court

terme sur le rat, bien que limitées, indiquent que dans les conditions
où se produit habituellement l'exposition humaine, il est peu
probable que le risque encouru soit très grave.

Une exposition par inhalation à une concentration de 15 220 mg/m^3
a affecté la fonction de reproduction de rats mâles, ce qui n'a pas
été le cas à la dose de 8610 mg/m^3. Chez des rattes gravides, la dose
sans effet observable se situait à 9001 mg/^{3} (3659 ppm); quant à la
dose la plus faible donnant lieu à un effet observable, elle était de
14 893 mg/m^3 (6054 ppm), en ce qui concerne la toxicité pour la
mère et le foetus. L'exposition par inhalation à de fortes
concentrations de propanol-1 a donc des effets nocifs sur la
reproduction et le développement des rats mâles et femelles
lorsque les concentrations utilisées sont manifestement toxiques
pour ces animaux. Pour obtenir ces effets, il a fallu utiliser des
concentrations plus élevées que celles auxquelles l'homme pourrait
être normalement exposé.

Différentes épreuves ont montré que le propanol-1 ne provoquait
pas de mutations ponctuelles chez les bactéries. Toutefois, si ces
résultats donnent à penser que le produit n'est pas génotoxique, les
données disponibles sont trop limitées pour qu'on puisse en évaluer
correctement le pouvoir mutagène. La seule étude dont on possède
les résultats ne permet pas d'évaluer convenablement la
cancérogénicité du propanol-1 chez l'animal d'expérience. On ne
dispose d'aucune donnée sur l'exposition à long terme des
populations humaines à ce produit, de sorte qu'on ne peut pas se
prononcer sur son pouvoir cancérogène chez l'homme.

A part un cas d'intoxication mortelle consécutif à l'ingestion d'un
demi-litre de propanol-1, il n'existe pratiquement aucun rapport
concernant d'éventuels effets nocifs découlant d'une exposition au
propanol-1, qu'il s'agisse de la population générale ou de groupes
professionnels. Le Groupe spécial estime qu'il est improbable que
le propanol-1 presente des risques graves pour la population
générale dans les conditions normales d'exposition.

Du propanol-1 peut être libéré dans l'environnement lors de la
production, de la transformation, du stockage, du transport, de
l'utilisation ou de rejet de ce produit. Comme il est essentiellement
utilisé comme solvant volatil, l'essentiel de la production finit par
aboutir dans l'atmosphère. Toutefois, par réaction avec les

radicaux hydroxyles et entraînement par les précipitations, le propanol-1 est rapidement éliminé de l'atmosphère, d'où il disparaît en moins de trois jours. Le propanol-1 s'élimine également rapidement de l'eau et du sol de sorte que l'on ne le rencontre que rarement en concentrations mesurables dans l'air, l'eau et la terre. Le propanol-1 est peu absorbé par les particules du sol où il se révèle mobile et dont il accroît la perméabilité à certains hydrocarbures aromatiques.

Compte tenu des propriétés physiques du propanol-1, il est peu probable qu'il donne lieu à une bioaccumulation et sauf accident ou rejet négligent, le propanol-1 ne présente aucun risque pour la faune ou la flore aquatique aux concentrations où on le rencontre habituellement dans l'environnement.

RESUMEN

1. Identidad, propiedades físicas y químicas, métodos analíticos

El 1-propanol es un líquido incoloro y sumamente inflamable, volátil a temperatura ambiente y presión atmosférica normal. Es miscible con el agua y los disolventes orgánicos. Entre los métodos analíticos para el propanol figuran la cromatografía de gases, que puede detectar hasta 5×10^{-5} mg/m^3 en el aire, $1\ 10^{-4}$ mg/litro en el agua y 0,002 mg/litro en la sangre, el suero o la orina cuando se utilizan con la muestra procedimientos adecuados de extracción o concentración.

2. Fuentes de exposición humana y ambiental

En 1979, la capacidad de producción mundial al año superó las 130 000 toneladas. En la naturaleza se produce por descomposición de material orgánico por diversos microorganismos, y se halla en las plantas y en los aceites combustibles. El 1-propanol se produce a partir del eteno por reacción con el monóxido de carbono y el hidrógeno para dar propionaldehído, que a continuación se hidrogena. Aparece también como subproducto en la fabricación del metanol y puede producirse a partir del propano directamente o a partir de la acroleína. El uso principal del 1-propanol es como disolvente de uso múltiple en la industria y el hogar. Se utiliza en las tintas de impresión flexográfica y en aplicaciones textiles, productos de uso personal como cosméticos y lociones, en productos para limpiar cristales, en abrillantadores y en fórmulas antisépticas. Le sigue en importancia su uso como producto intermedio en la fabricación de diversos compuestos químicos.

3. Transporte, distribución y transformación en el medio ambiente

La principal vía de entrada del 1-propanol en el medio ambiente es su emisión a la atmósfera durante la producción, el tratamiento, el almacenamiento, el transporte, el uso y la evacuación de desechos. También se producen emisiones al agua y al suelo. Puesto que el uso principal del 1-propanol es como disolvente volátil, gran parte del volumen de producción acaba en el medio ambiente.

El 1-propanol desaparece rápidamente de la atmósfera por reacción con radicales hidroxilo y por el lavado con la lluvia. Es fácilmente biodegradable, tanto en condiciones aerobias como anaerobias y, a causa de estos mecanismos de eliminación química y biológica, no suelen encontrarse niveles medibles de la sustancia en el medio ambiente. No obstante, se ha detectado en la atmósfera urbana, en vertederos de desechos y también en las aguas que se rezumaban de un terraplenado. La permeabilidad del suelo al 1-propanol es probablemente elevada y el compuesto aumenta la permeabilidad a ciertos disolventes aromáticos.

El 1-propanol tiene un coeficiente de reparto log n-octanol/agua de 0,34 y un factor de bioconcentración de 0,7, lo que hace muy poco probable su bioacumulación.

4. Niveles ambientales y exposición humana

La exposición de la población general puede producirse por ingestión accidental, por inhalación durante el uso y por ingestión junto con los alimentos (que contengan 1-propanol como aromatizante volátil natural o añadido o como residuo de disolvente) y bebidas alcohólicas y no alcohólicas. Por ejemplo, la cerveza contiene hasta 195 mg/litro, el vino hasta 116 mg/litro y los diversos tipos de licores hasta 3520 mg/litro. La exposición de la población general al 1-propanol por inhalación y en el agua de bebida es baja (en los Estados Unidos, la concentración media en muestras de aire urbano fue de 0,00005 mg/m^3 y la correspondiente al agua de bebida 0,001 mg/litro). Aunque los trabajadores están potencialmente expuestos por la inhalación durante la fabricación, el tratamiento y la utilización, no se dispone de datos para cuantificar esas exposiciones.

5. Cinética y metabolismo

El 1-propanol se absorbe y distribuye rápidamente por todo el organismo tras la ingestión. Se carece de datos sobre la tasa de absorción tras la inhalación y la exposición dérmica. El 1-propanol es metabolizado por la deshidrogenasa alcohólica para dar ácido propiónico por intermedio del aldehído y puede entrar en el ciclo del ácido tricarboxílico. Esta oxidación es una etapa limitativa de la velocidad del metabolismo del 1-propanol. *In vitro*, las oxidasas microsómicas de rata y conejo también son capaces de oxidar el 1-propanol a aldehído propiónico. La afinidad relativa de la deshidrogenasa alcohólica y los sistemas de oxidación microsómicos por el 1-propanol es mucho más elevada que en el caso del etanol; así pues, el 1-propanol se elimina rápidamente del organismo. En la rata, el periodo de semieliminación de una dosis oral de 1000 mg/kg fue de 45 minutos.

Tanto en animales como en el hombre, el 1-propanol puede ser eliminado del organismo en el aire exhalado o en la orina. A sujetos a los que se administró una dosis de 1-propanol de 3,75 mg por kg de peso corporal y 1200 mg de etanol por kg de peso corporal por vía oral, la excreción urinaria total de 1-propanol fue del 2,1% de la dosis. Los niveles urinarios de 1-propanol fueron más bajos cuanto más baja era la cantidad de etanol ingerida simultáneamente, lo que demuestra la competencia por la deshidrogenasa alcohólica entre el 1-propanol y la sobredosis de etanol.

6. Efectos en los organismos en el medio ambiente

A las concentraciones en que normalmente se encuentra en el medio ambiente, el 1-propanol no resulta tóxico para los organismos acuáticos, los insectos ni las plantas. El umbral de inhibición para la multiplicación celular de tres de las especies acuáticas más sensibles (tres protozoos) fue de 38–568 mg/litro. Para los organismos superiores, la concentración letal fue de unos 5000 mg/litro, y variaba notablemente poco de un filum a otro y exhibía una curva dosis-respuesta sumamente pronunciada. Algunas bacterias y microorganismos de aguas residuales y cienos activados son capaces de adaptarse a concentraciones superiores a 17 000 mg/litro.

La germinación de semillas puede verse inhibida o estimulada por el 1-propanol según la concentración en el agua utilizada y las condiciones de exposición. El compuesto aumenta la acumulación de nitritos en el maíz, los guisantes y el trigo.

7. Efectos en animales de experimentación y en sistemas de ensayo *in vitro*

La toxicidad aguda del 1-propanol para los mamíferos (a juzgar por la mortalidad) es baja, por cualquiera de las vías de exposición: cutánea, oral o respiratoria. Se ha comunicado que los valores de la DL_{50} por vía oral para varias especies animales varían entre 1870 y 6800 mg/kg de peso corporal. No obstante, en ratas muy jóvenes se notificó una DL_{50} por vía oral de 560–660 mg/kg de peso corporal. El principal efecto tóxico del 1-propanol tras una exposición única es la depresión del sistema nervioso central. Los datos de que se dispone sobre el 1-propanol parecen indicar que sus efectos sobre el sistema nervioso central son semejantes a los del etanol; no obstante, el 1-propanol parece ser más neurotóxico. Los valores de la DE_{50} para la narcosis en el conejo y la pérdida del reflejo de enderezamiento en el ratón fueron, respectivamente, de 1440 mg/kg de peso corporal por vía oral, y de 1478 mg/kg de peso corporal por vía intraperitoneal; estos valores son unas cuatro veces más bajos que los correspondientes al etanol. En el ensayo del plano inclinado, el 1-propanol fue 2,5 veces más potente que el etanol en la rata.

La administración de dosis únicas por vía oral de 3000 ó 6000 mg/kg de peso corporal tuvo como resultado una acumulación reversible de triglicéridos en el hígado de la rata. Las concentraciones elevadas de vapor provocaron irritaciones en el tracto respiratorio del ratón. El ritmo respiratorio del ratón se vio disminuido en un 50% a concentraciones de aproximadamente 30 000 mg/m^3.

No se dispone de datos sobre irritación ocular y cutánea. No se observó sensibilización en una prueba de sensibilización cutánea en ratones CF1.

En machos de rata expuestos durante seis semanas a 15 220 mg/m^3, se obtuvieron pruebas limitadas de que el 1-propanol disminuye la capacidad reproductora. No se observaron efectos tras una exposición similar a 8610 mg/m^3. Cuando se expusieron ratas gestantes al 1-propanol, se observó toxicidad materna y fetal a 23 968 y 14 893 mg/m^3 (9743 y 6054 ppm); no se observó toxicidad a 9001 mg/m^3 (3659 ppm). No se observaron defectos de comportamiento en la progenie de machos de rata expuestos durante seis semanas a 8610 ó 15 220 mg de 1-propanol/m^3, ni en la de ratas expuestas durante la gestación a las mismas concentraciones. No obstante, cuando se administró a ratas de 5 a 8 días de edad 3000–7800 mg de 1-propanol/kg por vía oral al día, se observó depresión del sistema nervioso central durante la dosificación y síntomas de privación cuando se retiraba la dosis. Cuando las ratas cumplieron 18 días se examinaron sus cerebros y se observaron reducciones en los pesos cerebrales absoluto y relativo y en el contenido de ADN, así como disminuciones regionales de los niveles de colesterol y de proteínas.

El 1-propanol dio resultados negativos en dos ensayos de detección de mutaciones puntuales utilizando *Salmonella typhimurium* y en un ensayo de mutación inversa realizado con *Escherichia coli* CA-274. Se obtuvieron resultados negativos en ensayos para inducir intercambio de cromátidas hermanas o micronúcleos en células de mamíferos *in vitro*. No se obtuvieron otros datos sobre mutagenicidad.

En un estudio de carcinogenicidad realizado en grupos reducidos de ratas Wistar expuestas durante toda su vida a dosis orales de 240 mg/kg o a dosis subcutáneas de 48 mg/kg, se observó un aumento significativo de la incidencia de sarcoma hepático en el grupo en el que la dosis se administraba por vía subcutánea. No obstante, el estudio resultó insuficiente para evaluar la carcino-genicidad por diversos motivos, entre ellos la falta de detalle experimental, el reducido número de animales y el empleo de una sola dosis elevada para inducir toxicidad hepática.

8. Efectos en la salud humana

No se tiene noticia de efectos adversos para la salud en la población general o en grupos profesionales. El único caso notificado de intoxicación mortal, fue el de una mujer que perdió el conocimiento y falleció a las 4–5 h de la ingestión. La autopsia reveló "inflamación cerebral" y edema pulmonar. En un estudio sobre irritación cutánea y sensibilización, se comunicó la aparición de reacciones alérgicas en un operario de laboratorio. En otro grupo de 12 voluntarios, se observó en 9 individuos un eritema que duró al menos 60 minutos tras la aplicación durante 5 minutos de papeles de filtro impregnados con 0,025 ml de una solución al 75% de 1-propanol en agua aplicados sobre los antebrazos. No se dispone de más informes sobre efectos adversos para la salud tras la exposición profesional al 1-propanol.

No se dispone de estudios epidemiológicos para evaluar los efectos a largo plazo, incluida la carcinogenicidad, del 1-propanol en el ser humano.

9. Resumen de la evaluación

La exposición del ser humano al 1-propanol puede producirse por la ingestión de alimentos o bebidas que lo contengan. La exposición por inhalación puede tener lugar durante el uso doméstico de la sustancia y en el ámbito laboral durante su fabricación, tratamiento y uso. Los muy limitados datos de que se dispone sobre el nivel de 1-propanol en el aire y el agua parecen indicar que las concentraciones son muy reducidas.

El 1-propanol se absorbe y distribuye rápidamente por todo el organismo tras la ingestión. Se cree que la absorción tras la inhalación es rápida y la absorción por vía cutánea lenta.

La toxicidad aguda del 1-propanol para los animales es baja en toda exposición, ya sea por vía cutánea, oral o respiratoria. La exposición de miembros de la población general a niveles potencialmente letales puede producirse por ingestión accidental o intencionada. No obstante, sólo se ha notificado un caso de envenenamiento mortal por 1-propanol. Los efectos agudos más probables del 1-propanol en el hombre son la intoxicación alcohólica y la narcosis. Los resultados de los estudios en animales indican que el 1-propanol es 2–4 veces más tóxico que el etanol.

El 1-propanol puede ser irritante para la piel hidratada.

Los datos sobre toxicidad animal no bastan para evaluar los riesgos para la salud humana asociados a la exposición repetida o duradera al 1-propanol. No obstante, estudios limitados a corto plazo sobre la rata indican que la exposición por vía oral al 1-propanol tiene pocas probabilidades de suponer un riesgo grave para la salud en las condiciones habituales de exposición humana.

En la rata la exposición por inhalación a una concentración de 15 220 mg/m^3 redujo la capacidad reproductiva del macho, pero no así la exposición a 8610 mg/m^3. En la rata gestante, 9001 mg/m^3

(3659 ppm) fue el nivel de efectos no observados y 14 893 mg/m^3 (6054 ppm) el nivel más bajo de observación de efectos tanto respecto a la toxicidad materna como a la fetal. Así pues, la exposición por inhalación a concentraciones elevadas de 1-propanol produjo toxicidad reproductiva y embriológica en el macho y la hembra en presencia de toxicidad manifiesta en los animales expuestos. Las concentraciones necesarias para producir esos efectos en la rata fueron más elevadas que las que probablemente se observen en condiciones normales de exposición humana.

El 1-propanol dio resultados negativos en los ensayos de detección de mutaciones puntuales en bacterias. Aunque esto indica que la sustancia no tiene ningún potencial genotóxico, no puede evaluarse adecuadamente la mutagenicidad basándose en los limitados datos disponibles. El estudio realizado no basta para evaluar la carcinogenicidad del 1-propanol en animales de experimentación. No se dispone de datos sobre la exposición a largo plazo de poblaciones humanas al 1-propanol. Por todo ello, no puede evaluarse la carcinogenicidad del 1-propanol en el ser humano.

Aparte de un caso de intoxicación mortal tras la ingestión de medio litro de 1-propanol, no se tiene prácticamente noticia de efectos adversos para la salud producidos por la exposición al 1-propanol, ni en la población general ni en grupos profesionales. El Grupo Especial de Trabajo considera poco probable que el 1-propanol plantee un riesgo grave para la salud de la población general en condiciones normales de exposición.

El 1-propanol puede liberarse al medio ambiente durante la producción, el tratamiento, el almacenamiento, el transporte, el uso y la evacuación de desechos. A causa de su uso principal como disolvente volátil, la mayoría del volumen de producción acaba por ser liberado a la atmósfera. No obstante, por reacciones con radicales hidroxilo y por lavado pluvial, el 1-propanol desaparecerá rápidamente de la atmósfera, siendo su tiempo de presencia en ella inferior a 3 días. La eliminación del 1-propanol del agua y del suelo también se produce rápidamente, de modo que raras veces se detectan niveles medibles en cualquiera de estos tres compartimientos. La adsorción del 1-propanol en las partículas del suelo es escasa, pero la sustancia es móvil en el suelo y se ha demostrado que aumenta la permeabilidad del mismo a ciertos hidrocarburos aromáticos.

En vista de las propiedades físicas del 1-propanol, la bio-acumulación es poco probable y, salvo en el caso de evacuación accidental o inadecuada, el 1-propanol no constituye un riesgo para los organismos acuáticos, los insectos y las plantas en las concentraciones que por lo general se encuentran en el medio ambiente.

www.ingramcontent.com/pod-product-compliance
Lightning Source LLC
Chambersburg PA
CBHW071723210326
41597CB00017B/2566